WHEN WORDS ARE NOT ENOUGH

BY

Lorrie C. Reed, PhD, MA, MTS

&

Mary E. Carey, PhD, APRN

WHEN WORDS ARE NOT ENOUGH

BY

LORRIE C. REED & MARY E. CAREY

Copyright © 2010   Allen Carey Associates LLC

ISBN 978-0-98296-290-9

All rights reserved. Printed in the United States of America.

No part of this publication may be reproduced, in any form or by any means, without the written consent of Allen Carey Associates LLC

    Contact: Allen Carey Associates LLC
                         P.O. Box 890053
                         Oklahoma City, OK 73189-0053
                         Telephone: 405-834-8279
                         Fax: 405-720-9924

TABLE OF CONTENTS

	Page Number
Preface…………………………………………………	4
Chapter One – Introduction……………………………..	7
Chapter Two – Theme One: Reflective Retrospection…….	13
Chapter Three – Theme Two: Positive Coping Strategies…	29
Chapter Four – Theme Three: Holism and Equilibrium……..	42
Chapter Five – Theme Four: Spiritual Discipline…………..	60
Chapter Six – Theme Five: Shared Wisdom………………	70
Chapter Seven – Summary and Resources…………………	77
Bibliography……………………………………………..	96

WHEN WORDS ARE NOT ENOUGH

BY

LORRIE C. REED, PhD, MA, MTS & MARY E. CAREY, PhD, APRN

"The most precious gift we can offer others is our presence. When our mindfulness embraces those we love they will bloom like flowers."

-- from Thich Nhat Hanh, *Living Buddha Living Christ*

Preface

Purpose of the Book

When Words Are Not Enough provides basic facts and suggests ways that caregivers might have an impact upon the holistic well-being of care recipients with Alzheimer's disease and other forms of dementia. A secondary purpose of this book is to suggest ways to help caregivers cope with the ongoing stress associated with their labor of love. This book will define, describe, and analyze issues concerning the needs of dementia caregivers. The analysis will be multifaceted and will give consideration to physiological, psychological, sociological, and spiritual aspects of the problem. For purposes of this discussion, a *caregiver* is defined as a healing facilitator, advocate, or other person who tends to the needs of someone who is unable to care for self. Our position is that we acknowledge the full humanity of all caregivers and will focus on remedies that nurture their empowerment, liberation, self-respect, and dignity.

As authors of this volume, we acknowledge our interpretive limitations as related to nationality, race, economic class, and age. Both of us are middle-aged, middle class, educated African American women who have lived and practiced in multicultural environments. Hence, our views are likely to be general with regard to the broader population but more specific in the context of the African American experience. When interpretive variations based on culture are deemed enlightening, pertinent details will be shared. We will approach the topic as objectively as possible given our cultural lenses.

This book is unique for a number of reasons. First of all it deals with caregivers' needs from a holistic frame of reference. Secondly, it targets caregivers of people who have been diagnosed with dementia of the Alzheimer's type and the professionals and paraprofessionals who care for them. Thirdly, Baby Boomers, in particular, will appreciate the holistic view embraced by the book. As this group continues to age, they will continue to care for their elders, their adult children, grandchildren, and each other.

Organization of the Book

Chapters in this book will touch upon a range of concerns, including a definition of dementia, an overview of current treatment of dementia patients, and a review of the needs of caregivers. Each chapter ends with a case study analysis. The book will end with a listing of resources and an extensive bibliography.

Objectives of This Book

1. Provide basic facts about dementia and Alzheimer's disease

2. Describe the disease's physical, psychological, and spiritual impact on the caregiver

3. Define holistic approaches to dealing with care recipients

4. Describe the disease's impact on interpersonal relationships

5. Describe compassion fatigue and caregivers' burden

6. Suggest ways for caregivers to engage in self-care

7. Provide resources to impact the well-being of caregivers

CHAPTER ONE - INTRODUCTION

Scope of the Problem

The American population is getting older. Recent life expectancy tables report that, "The number of people 60 or older will grow to nearly 2 billion in 2050, for the first time in recorded history outnumbering those who are younger than 15."[1] And within this segment of the population, the incidence of dementia and Alzheimer's disease is growing. It is estimated that Alzheimer's disease currently affects 2.4 million to 4.5 million Americans, many of whom fall into this age group. According to the Alzheimer's Foundation of America, the number of Americans with Alzheimer's disease could more than triple to 16 million by mid-century. As the number of care recipients increases, so will the number of caregivers. It is estimated that "one to four family members act as caregivers for each individual with Alzheimer's disease."[2]

Caring for people with dementia will become the responsibility of spouses or children. Providing caregivers with basic facts might have an impact upon the holistic well-being of care recipients with Alzheimer's disease and other forms of dementia. Such fundamental information may also prove to be helpful in decreasing the level of caregivers' burden.

Caregivers' Concerns

So many times, as caregivers, we feel frustration, resentment, unspecified stress, and weariness as we try to meet the needs of our aging loved ones. Having worked all our lives, we have looked forward to the days when we can rest from our labors and enjoy the benefits of retirement we so richly deserve. Often, however, our dreams may be delayed because our parents are mentally declining or physically ill. Just as they cared for us for so many years, their care now falls to us – their children, their caregivers, the baby boomers, and the sandwich generation. From time to time we find ourselves searching for answers but cannot lay our hands readily on the information we need to address our questions. Not only that, our uncertainty and anxiety are intensified because we are unaware of the challenges ahead, and frequently we don't even know what questions to ask. And then, often, we want to hear from or be reassured by someone who understands our plight. Where do we garner strength? Where do we find support? Where do we obtain the information we need?

Most of us have been touched in some way as our parents have grown older. This was the case for one of the authors of this book. Her father-in-law, who suffered from Alzheimer's disease along with a number of other severe physical ailments, was no longer able to care for himself, yet he wanted to remain in his home. The author and her husband had tried other care strategies such as checking on him frequently during the week and hiring a live-in, full-time, professional caregiver. None of these approaches, however, seemed to satisfy his needs. It quickly became apparent that it was time to consider a residential care arrangement. After talking to several agencies and visiting many assisted living facilities, the author and her husband concluded that a nursing home would be the best solution. They agonized over the decision, but in the end, the nursing home proved to be the best placement for him because of his health challenges. Predictably, his decline was gradual but inevitable. Seeing him in his diminished state caused both the author and her husband to sink into deep sadness from time to time when they went to visit him. Dad used to embody such a vital and commanding presence. After disease began to compromise his well-being, he exuded only a glimmer of that former self. The author and her husband were overwhelmed by their lack of understanding of Dad's diseases.

This author's great grandmother was also touched by Alzheimer's. For her, the disease prompted a constant search for a state of peace she had experienced in her younger years in Mississippi. To hear her tell it, against her will, she had been forced to travel with her family to Chicago during the Great Migration. Yet her heart remained in Clarksdale, and she was determined to get back there one day. On restless days, she perseverated on collecting her belongings -- a few pieces of clothing, an inexpensive broach, and a few faded photographs, which she bundled up in a big floral kerchief. She didn't remember much about what was going on around her from one minute to the next. For example, she could never distinguish me from my sister; nor could she recall whether or not she'd had eggs or cereal for breakfast. But she always remembered to put on her hat. And she remembered with astonishing clarity which direction was south. Oh yes, we all knew the pattern. When she went missing all we had to do is follow her trail southward toward the only home she remembers, the place where she found peace.

Then there was the experience with this author's step-grandmother. Her wails were incessant, high-pitched, and heart rending. As she grew older, she was no longer able to tend to her own increasingly demanding physical needs. And dementia had started to set in. So her son and stepdaughter took her in and put her up in the best guest room their house had to offer. It was neat and clean and adorned with cheerful motifs that would bring a smile to just about anyone's face. But she didn't notice. She was consumed with loneliness and mistrust, and she longed to be back in her own house where she had lived for more than 70 years. Nothing except Akron would be good enough, for her real home was where the memories were.

In the situations described above, caregivers' burden becomes a matter of concern. According to a recent article, caring for a loved one in the home presents special challenges and stressors for the dementia caregiver. The physical, financial, and emotional challenges often seem to be overwhelming. To complicate matters, the well-being of the caregiver has an impact on the survival and quality of life of the dementia care recipient. The article notes: "An overwhelmed caregiver can result in premature institutionalization and increased health-care utilization, by both the patients and the caregivers."[3] For this reason, physicians are cautioned to assess caregivers periodically for the:

"level of perceived burden, presence of depression and anxiety, social support, behavioral problems in the care recipient, and coping strategies and help the patient and caregiver with advance care planning. Strategies that meld support, education, and practical counseling about common caregiving stresses and community resources seem to mitigate caregiver burden and depression." [4]

Survey of Caregivers' Needs

As a way of increasing our understanding and awareness of issues pertaining to caregivers' burden, the authors of this book invited 14 relatives of chronically ill, older adults to take part in a non-scientific, informal, anonymous survey to assess caregivers' needs. Participation consisted of completing a demographic profile, answering three open-ended questions, and providing responses to short inventories. Information was collected through use of an on-line data gathering tool entitled the "Holistic Fitness for Caregivers Survey." The majority of respondents were between 45 and 65 (n=11) years of age, were female (n=11) and African American (n=13). Approximately 50% were married (n=7) and cared for the care recipient in their home (n=6). Nine caregivers were employed outside of the home, and the vast majority had an educational level ranging from some college to beyond a master's degree. Approximately 50% of the caregivers were also helping to meet the needs of their children (n=6).

The nature of the care recipients' illnesses included dementia, cancer, stroke, and the general category of "other." The majority of caregivers had served in that role for five years or less. The amount of time spent in the caregiver role ranged from less than six hours per week (n=3) to six to 10 hours per week (n=6). Eleven hours to over 20 hours of caregiving per week were expended by several respondents (n=5).

Five major themes emerged from the survey data.

1. There is value in the exercise of reflective retrospective analysis of the caregiving role.

2. Caregiving influences the equilibrium of familial and non-familial social systems.

3. Positive coping strategies used by caregivers are valuable tools.

4. Spiritual discipline can ease the strain of caregiving.

5. Seasoned caregivers have caregiving wisdom to share with others.

In addition to responding to general demographic data, respondents shared valuable insights and practical wisdom in their answers to several open-ended items. Each of the five themes that emerged will be explored in greater detail in the chapters that follow.

Chapter Two – Theme One: Reflective Retrospection

Theme Summary

Theme 1: There is value in the exercise of reflective retrospective analysis of the caregiving role.

A common thread running through survey comments was the need for up-to-date, accurate information about the disease, the physical and emotional needs of the care recipient, and the quality and responsibility of the care facilities involved. These concerns indicate that an informational component is associated with meeting the needs of caregivers. This need for information grows out of retrospective reflection about the caregiving situation.

Survey Responses

Participants were asked to think about the time when they first became a caregiver and to respond to the following probe: "If I knew then what I know now, I would..." One participant said:

"If I knew then what I know now I would have pushed harder to get information regarding home services and programs from social workers at the hospital and rehab center. I would have fought even harder so that my mother could receive more benefits and equipment instead of taking someone's word for it. I would have pushed the homecare therapists and my mother to work harder on her recovery much sooner. I honestly would have looked into going after the hospital for neglect so that she [could] be afforded the best equipment and home care, not just what we can do. I should have fought more people along the way instead of saying okay when [others] told [me] that's just the way it is."

Another respondent noted the need to have immediate, accurate information about the disease:

"My husband and I would have recognized the symptoms of [Alzheimer's] earlier. By the time we actually realized what was going on Dad was in the second stage. He had developed ways of coping with his illness that weren't exactly healthy. We initially tried a live-in caregiving service, but that didn't work out. So we ended up placing him in a nursing home. Thinking back on it, I can now recall tell-tale signs of the disease. But those signs didn't add up until much later. It often makes me wonder what would have happened if we had detected the disease earlier."

Having information about options for home care and assistance with daily routines was a need expressed by another participant:

"I would have contacted a social service agency for a home care provider (non-medical) to assist with some of the daily routine tasks. Full-time employment is draining if you are a dedicated worker; having additional responsibilities placed a lot of additional stress on me and my other sibling who was also working full time."

Knowing how to support the loved one physically and emotionally was a concern expressed by another participant.

"[I would] not have spoiled my mother. Feeling sorry for someone (my mother) because you love them so much, I realized I did not help her. Now, she does not want to do anything for herself, little things like walking for exercises, fixing her own plate, or giving herself a shower. I don't want to hurt her feelings, especially when she gets so irritated when she can't remember anything that just happened recently."

Having information about not only the symptoms of the disease but also the responsibilities of care facilities was a need expressed by another participant.

"[I would have] paid more attention to symptoms; been more patient with my mother; stayed on top of healthcare professionals, particularly hospital staff and nursing home staff. In most cases, service/care was abominable. Nursing home care was criminal neglect. I would also have dealt very differently with 'family stuff.' Situations like this can bring out the best, but also can bring out the WORST in people."

Relevant Academic Literature

As reflected in the comments above, the caregiver assumes more and more responsibility for care as patients begin to decline. This tendency is reinforced by recent academic research, which indicates that what used to be a "two-way dyadic patient–physician relationship ... changes to a three-way relationship that includes the physician, the patient, and the family caregiver."[5] This, of course, heightens the importance of communication that addresses the needs and concerns of both the care recipient as well as the caregiver. A research study by Schulman and Hanson addresses this issue in part. During interviews conducted as part of their study caregivers were asked whether the nursing home care recipient needed more treatment or care from staff than they received for a specific symptom. Interviewees indicated that "30% of dying nursing home residents needed more care for emotional and spiritual needs, 23% needed more care to ensure personal cleanliness, and 19% needed more treatment for pain."[6] In a research study conducted by Liebert, participating caregivers perceived that the clinical care provided by the staff of nursing homes to their loved ones was poor and often neglectful. The study concluded that "caregivers who were concerned about these issues perceived overall communication as particularly poor,"[7] leaving caregivers with the impression that health care providers were hiding something.

In a study conducted by Sanders et al., the daughter of a care recipient indicated that she felt as if she were fighting the system. She did not feel that the instructions and preferences she specified for her loved one were being taken seriously, thereby causing both the caregiver and recipient high levels of distress.[8] In this same study, the wife of a care recipient expressed her frustration. She reported that:

"My husband just had pneumonia and he couldn't talk and tell them what he needed. So, I was there . . . one day it was ten hours, the next day it was nine. Just to be there and be the advocate for these people. He called the nurses in and fifteen minutes later they came in and he ended up getting up from the bed and peeing on the floor on the way to the bathroom. She [nurse] was saying some really bad things to him; terms that were not very nice."[9]

The wife further reported that during this hospital stay, the nurses did not take the time to toilet her husband and change his bed after episodes of incontinence. Consequently, the nurses left her husband naked in an unmade bed on frequent occasions.

The Sanders et al. study further indicates that case management and social services were not available at this facility when assistance was needed or when answers were sought. Not only that; professionals responsible for patient care did not return phone calls. Upon contacting the local chapter of the Alzheimer's Association, one caregiver spoke with four different people and received four different answers. As it turned out, none of the answers were correct. Eager to obtain answers, this caregiver also contacted an agency that had announced having volunteers available to help older adults. The caregiver was very disappointed to learn that, in fact, no volunteers were available.[10]

Other caregivers expressed feelings of frustration related to not being able to obtain needed information and services, lack of confidence in the dementia-related knowledge of many of the health care professionals, and feelings that they were being "shuffled from one person to the next without being able to get needed services or information."[11] One study reported that:

"All of these experiences created stress that could have been prevented through the provision of more informed, sensitive care to patients and their families. Although these experiences may be true for caregivers at any stage of the disease process and with any level of grief, these experiences seemed to magnify the grief of the caregivers in this study."[12]

Implications for Caregivers

Caregivers need accurate, up-to-date information to support their decisions.

What is dementia?
Dementia is defined as "the loss of mental processing ability, including communication, abstract thinking, judgment and physical abilities, such that it interferes with daily living."[13] The disease is associated with limited judgment, decreased memory, physical losses, and decline in environmental awareness – all of which limit communication. People with dementia are especially vulnerable, the research notes, to being lonely and bewildered, grieving or desperately trying to communicate. Moreover, Goldsmith reports that "they are almost certainly frightened at some stage in their illness."[14] When presented with a diagnosis of dementia, the health care delivery

17

system supports a disease management model and seeks a medical diagnosis. The DSMIV-TR presents the following criteria for dementia.

"Although classified as mental disorders due to deterioration in mental, behavioral, and emotional functioning, all these brain disorders are probably caused by physical disease, trauma or the effects of drugs and are classified according to the underlying disease state."[15]

A diagnosis for a client who has been experiencing fluctuating states of health can be a comfort to the care recipient and the caregiver whether they are familial or non-familial, professional or paraprofessional, compensated or volunteer. However, in all situations, the caregiver responds directly to symptoms of the disease entity or diagnosis. The management of these symptoms can be particularly challenging for the lay caregiver. It is estimated that 24 million Americans are living with some form of dementia.[16]

It is important to note here that dementia needs to be distinguished from delirium, a frequently reversible cognitive state. The DSM-IV-TR presents the following criteria for delirium: Unlike dementia, delirium involves fluctuating levels of consciousness and pervasive impairment in mental, behavioral, and emotional functioning. Delirium usually is of acute onset and temporary duration. Similar to dementia, delirium is probably caused by physical disease, head trauma, or the effect of drugs.[17]

What is Alzheimer's Disease?
Alzheimer's disease, a form of dementia, is a progressive and fatal brain disease that destroys brain cells, causing problems with memory and thinking. It is the most

common form of dementia and causes memory loss and impairment of other intellectual abilities. More than 5 million Americans have been affected by Alzheimer's disease in recent years.[18] Although support and services have been shown to contribute to a better life for people living with Alzheimer's disease, modern science has not yet found a cure. Tragically, Alzheimer's disease gets worse over time. Symptoms are treatable, but eventually, the disease results in fatal malfunctioning of the body's nerve-cell networks. While support and services can make life better for people living with Alzheimer's, the disease is fatal.[19]

People with Alzheimer's disease present symptoms that caregivers should recognize. Among these symptoms are states of confusion, memory loss, impaired judgment, and impaired affect. Understanding the symptoms of the disease will benefit both caregivers and care recipients. We are indebted to the Alzheimer's Association for providing much of the information pertaining to these symptoms.

States of Confusion
It is very common for caregivers to verbally attempt to orient the confused care recipient to the parameters of time, place, and person. In other words, we often try to move the care recipient into our frame of logic. Caregivers need to keep in mind that such states of confusion are frequently not logical. The task of the caregiver is to connect with the care recipient. That could mean orientation to time, place, and person, or it could simply mean being supportive in the presence of the person being cared for.

Memory Loss
In the past, people believed that memory loss was a normal part of aging. They often regarded Alzheimer's disease as natural age-related decline. Experts now recognize severe memory loss as a symptom of serious illness, according to

the Alzheimer's Association.[20] At the same time, researchers have concluded that the question is still open as to whether memory naturally declines to some extent. Many people feel that their memory becomes less sharp as they grow older, but determining whether there is any scientific basis for this belief is a research challenge still being addressed. Under normal circumstances, aging adults tend to forget names or appointments occasionally. In the Alzheimer's patient, however, memory loss may involve forgetting recently learned information or the inability to later recall recently learned information. Remote memory is the last function to be eroded in the case of several irreversible dementias. Consequently, as caregivers, we should take advantage of that fact by supporting the memory function that remains with, for example, treatments such as reminiscence therapy via music and photographs.[21]

Impaired Judgment
Have you occasionally walked into a room and forgotten why you were there? Or have you opened your mouth and forgotten what you planned to say? These behaviors are normal for aging adults. Alzheimer's patients, on the other hand, experience difficulty performing familiar tasks or in planning and completing everyday tasks. For example, they often lose track of the steps involved in preparing a meal, placing a telephone call, or playing a game. Hence, monitoring of the care recipient is a very important function for the caregiver. Areas for particular concern relate to activities of daily living (i.e. bathing, dressing, and grooming). Gentle reminders of what is socially acceptable can be managed with verbal and non-verbal cues.[22]

Alzheimer's patients also experience poor or decreased judgment. This may involve dressing inappropriately, wearing several layers on a warm day or little clothing in the cold. Showing poor judgment may also entail things like giving away large sums of money to telemarketers or inappropriate use of the gas burners on a cooking stove. On the other hand, for people without Alzheimer's disease, making a questionable or debatable decision from time to time is normal.

Problems with abstract thinking or having unusual difficulty performing complex mental tasks may present themselves as warning signs of Alzheimer's. This might involve the aging person's forgetting what numbers are for and how they should be used. Normally, aging people might find it challenging to balance a checkbook.

Having problems with language may be another warning sign of Alzheimer's disease. Although it is quite normal for a person to have trouble finding the right word to express an idea or feeling, things like forgetting simple words or substituting unusual words may raise a red flag. For example, the Alzheimer's patient might ask for "that thing for my mouth" instead of asking specifically for a toothbrush.[23]

Misplacing things is another warning sign. Misplacing keys or a wallet temporarily can be considered normal behaviors. It may also be normal to forget the day of the week or where you were going. But putting things in unusual places, such as placing an iron in the freezer or a wristwatch in the sugar bowl, may be a warning sign for Alzheimer's disease. Another warning sign might be disorientation to time and place. For example, Alzheimer's patients might become lost in their own neighborhood. Or they might forget where they are, how they got there, and how to get back home.

Impaired Affect
Feeling sad or moody occasionally is normal behavior for most people. But impaired affect is part of the disease process. Consequently, consistency of affect on the part of the caregiver, predictability of routine, genuineness, and positive regard for the care recipient are very therapeutic communication tools. Impaired affect may involve changes in mood or behavior or showing rapid mood swings – from calmness to tears to anger – for no apparent reason.

Changes in personality may also represent impairment of the affect. Showing dramatic changes in personality, becoming extremely confused, suspicious, fearful, or dependent on a family member are all symptoms of this impairment. By comparison, under normal circumstances, most people have a tendency to undergo minor personality changes with age.

We all have had days when we feel weary of work or uninterested in fulfilling social obligations. This is normal. On the other hand, the Alzheimer's patient may experience loss of initiative or extreme passiveness. This may involve sitting in front of the television for hours, sleeping more than usual, or not wanting to do usual activities.[24]

Debunking Common Myths
It is important that caregivers distinguish myth from fact. The Alzheimer's Association has identified a number of these myths, clarified erroneous information, and made the facts widely available to the public. A number of their findings are presented in this section.[25]

At one time it was generally believed that only older people could get Alzheimer's disease. Researchers now know that this is not the case. Alzheimer's can strike people in their thirties, forties, and fifties. Of the more than 5 million Americans living with this debilitating disease, some 500,000 people under age 65 have Alzheimer's or a related disorder.

Another myth promotes the view that Alzheimer's disease is not fatal. In reality, Alzheimer's disease kills its victims. It destroys brain cells and causes memory changes, erratic behaviors, and loss of body functions. It slowly and painfully takes away the victims' identity, ability to connect with others, and even their ability to think, eat, talk, walk, and find their way home.

During the 1960s and 1970s, aluminum emerged as a possible cause of Alzheimer's. A widespread belief was that cooking in aluminum pots and pans or drinking out of aluminum cans could lead to onset of the disease. This suspicion led to concern about exposure to aluminum through everyday sources such as pots and pans, beverage cans, antacids, and antiperspirants. Since then, studies have failed to confirm any role for aluminum in causing Alzheimer's. Experts today focus on other areas of research, and few believe that everyday sources of aluminum pose any threat.

Aspartame had also been blamed for memory loss. This myth was later debunked. This artificial sweetener, marketed under a variety of brand names, was approved by the U.S. Food and Drug Administration (FDA) for use in all foods and beverages in 1996. Since approval, concerns about aspartame's health effects have been raised. According to the FDA, as of May 2006, the agency had not been presented with any scientific evidence that would lead the agency to change its conclusions on the safety of aspartame for most people. The agency says its conclusions are based on more than 100 laboratory and clinical studies.

Another common myth was that flu shots increased the risk of Alzheimer's disease. Research has shown that this is not the case. Although a theory linking flu shots to a greatly increased risk of Alzheimer's disease has been proposed by a U.S. doctor whose license was suspended by the South Carolina Board of Medical Examiners, new evidence has emerged. Several mainstream studies now link flu shots and other vaccinations to a reduced risk of Alzheimer's disease and overall better health.

Silver dental fillings also were thought to increase the risk of Alzheimer's disease. However, according to the best available scientific evidence, there is no relationship between silver dental fillings and Alzheimer's. The concern that there could be a link arose because "silver" fillings are made of an amalgam (mixture) that typically contains about 50% mercury, 35% silver, and 15% tin. Mercury is a heavy metal that, in certain forms, is known to be toxic to the brain and other organs. Public health agencies, including the FDA, the U.S. Public Health Service, and the World Health Organization, endorse the continued use of amalgam as safe, strong, inexpensive material for dental restorations.

A final myth is that there are treatments available to stop the progression of Alzheimer's disease. This, too, is untrue. At this time, there is no treatment to cure, delay, or stop the progression of Alzheimer's disease, although research is ongoing. FDA-approved drugs temporarily slow worsening of symptoms for about 6 to 12 months, on average, for about half of the individuals who take them.

Stages of Alzheimer's
Several methods exist to identify the various stages of Alzheimer's disease. The Alzheimer's Association identifies a seven-stage model. Other organizations describe only three stages to the disease. Regardless of the number of increments used to pinpoint progression of the disease, all of the models are similar in that they are based on symptoms linked to the degeneration of the brain and nervous system of Alzheimer's care recipients. The various systems provide helpful guidelines for understanding how the disease may develop. By the same token, caregivers should keep in mind that each individual progresses differently. Overlap exists in the cognitive, physical and functional phases of the disease in different care recipients. Moreover, the time associated with each stage varies widely, and not all patients experience all symptoms.

Early Stage - Alzheimer's (Mild)

Memory loss or other cognitive deficits are noticeable, yet the Alzheimer's patient can compensate for them and continue to function independently. The early stage of Alzheimer's disease is when problems with memory, thinking, and concentration may begin to appear in a doctor's interview or medical tests. Individuals in the early stage typically need minimal assistance with simple daily routines. At the time of a diagnosis, an individual is not necessarily in the early stage of the disease; he or she may have progressed beyond this phase. Communication is affected during this stage of Alzheimer's disease; dementia caregivers may find that increased concentration is required for the care recipient to follow conversations. Care recipients may also have trouble staying on topic. More time may be required for the care recipient to formulate verbal responses to questions due to difficulty in finding the right words at times. In addition, the care recipient may lose the train of thought more often than before symptoms began. In the process, both the caregiver and the care recipient may experience increased frustration.

Midstage - Alzheimer's (Moderate)

Mental abilities decline, the personality changes, and physical problems develop so that the person becomes more and more dependent on caregivers. The middle stage is marked by the care recipient's experiencing difficulty in understanding long conversations, difficulty understanding reading material, and difficulty finishing sentences. The care recipient may also have trouble explaining abstract concepts and may speak in vague and rambling sentences. Decreased ability to interpret facial expressions and inability to raise or lower the voice are also characteristic of this stage. All of this may result in apathy on the part of the care recipient, including reduced interest in communication.

Late stage - Alzheimer's (Severe)

Complete deterioration of the personality and loss of control over bodily functions requires total dependence on others for even the most basic activities of daily living. Care recipients in the late stage will show inability to understand the meaning of most words and will have problems realizing when they are being addressed. There may be diminished use of proper grammar. In some cases, the care recipient may become totally mute.

END OF CHAPTER EXERCISES
Caregiving When the Care Receiver Lives Alone

The case will focus on distance caregiving where the responsible relatives (distance) hire someone locally to offer the care.

Vignette: Mr. Smith, age 68, has been given an early diagnosis of Alzheimer's disease yet lives alone in his own home in a small rural town in the Southwest U.S. His only living daughter lives in the Midwest U.S. with her husband, teenage son, and daughter. She has been coordinating his care at a distance for the last 6 months with the help of a reliable home health care agency. She talks with her father on a daily basis and has recently noticed behaviors indicative of significant cognitive decline. Physically he continues to function within normal limits to the best of her knowledge.

Case Study Analysis Questions

1. Define the nature of the problem.
2. Use specific details that provide sufficient background for analysis.
3. Evaluate the seriousness of the problem.
4. Determine the extent to which some kind of action is required immediately.
5. Identify two or more alternative solutions.
6. Describe a particular course of action and describe your rationale for selecting it.
7. Describe a plan to implement the action you selected.

Chapter Three – Theme Two: Positive Coping Strategies

Theme Summary

Theme 2: Positive coping strategies used by caregivers are valuable tools.

Participants' comments indicated a physical component to coping with the burden of caregiving. This also involved relieving stress through physical mechanisms. Attending to physical health ensured that the caregiver had enough strength and stamina to thrive. Physical remedies also required the caregiver to get enough nourishment, exercise, release of tension, and rest.

Survey Responses

One section of the survey asked participants to respond to items about their coping strategies. Table I summarizes those responses.

A number of participants provided descriptions of steps they took to relax. One participant attended Curves at least three times per week or walked two to three miles when she was unable to attend Curves. This participant further reported that she relaxed by spending time engaging in the activities of "several social and professional organizations."

Table 1: Preferred Coping Strategies

\multicolumn{3}{c}{Preferred Coping Strategies}		
\multicolumn{3}{l}{Place a check mark in the space that indicates your level of agreement with each statement. Answer each question as it applies to your situation within the past 12 months. Use the following scale: 1 = Strongly Disagree, 2 = Disagree, 3 = Agree, 4 = Strongly Agree}		
Strategy	*Number of Responses*	*Rating Score*
I exercise at least once a month.	14	2.7
I consider myself to be a spiritual person.	14	3.7
I do leisurely reading at least once a week.	14	3.4
I work until I am exhausted on most days.	14	2.4
I pray at least once a day.	14	3.2
I find time for play at least once a week.	14	2.9

Another participant spoke about maintaining balance among her various responsibilities:

"I maintained a balance between my responsibilities to my mother, my then teen-aged child, and myself. At one point during the caregiver stage of my life I was also primary caregiver for my sister. My daughter was able to often make the visits to my sister. My sister actually enjoyed my daughter's visits better than those made by me. She would take her high school friends with her. This provided my

sister with an opportunity to find out what was taking place in my daughter's and her friends' lives."

Still another participant, who reported being an introvert, described that her relaxation activities involved taking time to herself: "to think, reflect, sleep, [and] walk along the lake. Also, during this time I was in school and that was a wonderful diversion."

Relevant Academic Literature

Positive coping strategies emerged as a strong component of self-care in related research studies. One study reports that "self-care can take the form of reconnecting with family and friends, time alone (for quiet contemplation, playing a sport, recreational reading, nature walking, etc.), community service, or religious practice."[26] Dang and his colleagues[27] provide a number of tips to help caregivers cope with stress.

They advise caregivers to educate themselves and then to take action. It is important that caregivers focus on self-care by maintaining leisure activities and enhancing social support, which may come from family, friends, or community resources. In addition, caregivers should learn to communicate openly with health care professionals and to adjust their expectations as the disease progresses. And finally, they should remember that there is no such thing as a "perfect caregiver." [28]

Dealing with unresolved feelings of grief was also shown to be a positive coping strategy. In a study investigating the impact of grief among Alzheimer's caregivers, Sanders, Ott, Kelber, and Noonan reported that when interacting with the social service and health care delivery systems, many caregivers encountered obstacles. This was especially prevalent among caregivers with high levels of grief. According to Sanders et al., "The caregivers felt that professionals were unaware of the emotional ... needs of the care recipient. The actions of these professionals created more anguish and grief because of the adverse impact that it did or could have on the care recipient."[29]

Even so, caregivers were able to identify coping strategies they used to help manage their grief. In one research article, caregivers defined the importance of animals in their lives. For some caregivers, the unconditional support of a pet fortified their ability to cope. These caregivers viewed their pets as companions that helped them counterbalance feelings of loneliness and isolation. Pets were also important to care recipients. Caregivers said that "the love that the care recipient had for [an] animal was important to remember, particularly after the care recipient moved to a long-term care facility."[30]

Sanders et al. suggested that caregivers experiencing high levels of grief may benefit from using professional support. These coping strategies are based on reducing feelings of isolation, decreasing perceived lack of freedom, and reducing guilt and regret while at the same time addressing feelings of loss. The strategies facilitate the building of networks and include such activities as attendance at support groups, educational programs, family meetings and counseling.[31] Moreover, the activities described here can help caregivers obtain additional information about the disease and discover ways to stay connected with the care recipient.[32]

Implications for Caregivers

Coping with caregivers' burden involves self-care.

Compassion fatigue

Empathic connection with one's clients is essential to the therapeutic relationship. However, repeatedly engaging with distressed clients may cause "compassion fatigue," a phenomenon characterized as feeling overwhelmed by experiencing the clients' suffering. Compassion fatigue can include the symptoms of post-traumatic stress disorder (PTSD). It is also a Secondary Traumatic Stress Disorder and refers to a gradual lessening of compassion over time. Compassion fatigue is common among victims of trauma and individuals who work directly with victims of trauma.[33]

The management of compassion fatigue is very challenging for professional and paraprofessional caregivers, as well as for familial and non-familial caregivers. The major categories of compassion fatigue are mental, physical, and social. Mental fatigue can be manifested by decreased concentration, temporary short-term memory loss, and depression. Physical fatigue is frequently manifested by disruption of biorhythms and changes in eating habits. Social fatigue is frequently manifested by the perceived loss of joy for normally enjoyable activities and/or isolation. The benefits of preventing compassion fatigue are obvious, "You can't take care of anyone else until you take care of yourself." The following articles are representative of the existing literature focusing on compassion fatigue.

A descriptive study by Holst, Lundgren, Olsen, and Ishoy is based upon two cases from an end-of-life care setting in Denmark, where dysfunctional family dynamics presented added challenges to the staff members in their efforts to provide optimal palliative care.[34] The hospice triad--the patient, the staff member and the family member--forms the basis for communication and intervention in a hospice. Higher expectations and demands of younger, more well-informed patients and family members often challenge hospice staff in terms of information and communication when planning for care. The inherent risk factors of working with patients in the terminal phase of life become a focal point in preventing the development of compassion fatigue among staff members. The article presents a series of coping strategies to more optimally manage dysfunctional families in a setting where time is of the essence. These coping strategies seek to empower the hospice team, to prevent splitting among staff members, and to improve quality of care.

There are several potential benefits of including rituals and healing practices into the hospice care setting for staff.[35] Evidence suggests that not only does it provide an outlet for hospice workers to express their grief and reflect on their work in an accepting environment thereby providing closure for their patient's passing but it has also been shown to decrease the risk of burnout and compassion fatigue. This article discusses the important aspects of grief rituals and provides an illustrative example of one such ritual.

The experience of compassion fatigue is an expected and common response to the professional task of routinely caring for children at the end of life.[36] Symptoms of compassion fatigue often mimic trauma reactions. Implementing strategies that span personal, professional, and organizational domains can help protect health care providers from the damaging effects of compassion fatigue. Providing pediatric palliative care within a constructive and supportive team can help caregivers deal with the relational challenges of compassion fatigue. Finally, any consideration of the toll of providing pediatric palliative care must be balanced with a consideration of the parallel experience of compassion satisfaction.

Health outcomes and, in particular, patient health outcomes have become a driving force within health-care delivery.[37] Little emphasis has been placed on the potential health consequences for nurses providing care and caring within the health-care system. Compassion fatigue (or secondary traumatic stress) has emerged as a natural consequence of caring for clients who are in pain, suffering, or traumatized. This paper sheds light on how nursing work might impact the health of nurses by exploring the concept of compassion fatigue. Limitations of current instruments to measure compassion fatigue are highlighted, and suggestions for future direction are presented.

The mental health of the returning peacekeeper parallels that of his or her partner. Partners of traumatized soldiers report more posttraumatic stress disorder symptoms, somatic and sleep problems, negative social support, and low marital morale than partners of non-traumatized soldiers. These indicators are consistent with systemic traumatology theory.[38] This comment traces the historical and theoretical foundations that underlie the concept of secondary trauma (i.e., compassion fatigue) and discusses the implications for family psychology practice in helping veterans and their families recover from their ordeals.

Recognizing the growing numbers of family therapists who are choosing a focus on death, dying, and bereavement, this next article addresses the nature of the commitment required--as well as the gifts and challenges presented by work in this area.[39] Particular attention is given to therapists' vulnerability to compassion fatigue and/or vicarious tramatization, both of which are described and discussed. A variety of strategies for individuals and institutions aimed at supporting professionals and preventing problems are considered. It is concluded that, as family therapists focus on self-care as well as client care, they have the potential to increase not only their effectiveness but also to enhance their own well-being. Implications for training and for research on this topic also are considered.

A literature review by Collins explores how interacting with seriously traumatized people has the potential to affect health-care workers.[40] The review begins with an introduction to posttraumatic stress disorder as being one of the possible negative consequences of exposure to traumatic events. The report proceeds with examining the concepts of vicarious tramatization, secondary traumatic stress, traumatic counter-transference, burnout and compassion fatigue, as potential adverse consequences for workers who strive to help people who are traumatized. The differences between these concepts are also discussed. The notion of compassion satisfaction is examined as findings have demonstrated that it is a protective factor which can be used as a buffer to prevent the aforementioned concepts. Conversely, findings have shown that a history of previous stressful life events in helpers is a potential risk factor. The review concludes with an overview of the concepts considered, but cautions against generalization of the findings owing to the dearth of longitudinal studies into the issues raised and also the lack of investigation into the many different types of trauma.

Salston and Figley[41] focus on the consequences for providers of working with survivors of traumatic events, particularly criminal victimization. The paper reviews the relevant research and treatment literature associated with secondary traumatic stress (STS) and related variables (burnout, compassion fatigue, vicarious trauma, and counter-transference). The latter part of the paper identifies the most important mitigating factors in the development of STS. These include good training specific to trauma work, a personal history of trauma, and the interpersonal resources of the worker. Implications for treatment, prevention, and research are discussed.[42]

Caregivers' Burden
The term *caregivers' burden* describes the physical, emotional, and financial strain of providing care. This phenomenon has been studied extensively in recent years, and various tests have been designed to measure levels of stress that caregivers experience.[43] Caregivers have been described as "hidden victims" of Alzheimer's disease.[44] Those who give ongoing care to the elderly generally experience two types of stress, namely, primary and secondary. According to Alzheimer's Solutions, everyday caregiving duties produce primary stress. Primary caregiving stress can be generated by such things as planning and implementing daily care for the care recipient, restraining the care recipient for safety reasons, helping the care recipient with bathing and toileting, or devising ways to manage difficult behavior such as agitation or wandering. On the other hand, secondary caregiving stress is associated with things like caregiver conflicts with other family members, economic hardships such as lost wages,

and restrictions on the caregiver's personal leisure and social activities. [45]

Parks and Novielli report that "By the year 2030, an estimated 20 percent of the U.S. population will be 65 years or older. As the American population ages, a growing number of people will be serving as caregivers for family members affected by dementia and other types of functional impairment. ... In day-to-day practice, family physicians are likely to see patients who serve as caregivers. In fact, one study of patients in a family practice demonstrated that 21 percent of the patients had caregiving responsibilities for persons with chronic medical conditions."[46] Other research reports that dementia caregivers are almost twice as likely to suffer from symptoms of depression and from chronic illness when compared with caregivers of patients without dementia.[47] They conclude that: "Almost all caregivers of dementia patients (90%) have some degree of burden."[48]

Dang et al. tend to confirm this idea that depression adds to the burden among caregivers. They report that a burdened caregiver is more likely to be depressed and to experience other medical problems. They further suggest that a high level of caregivers' burden may be responsible for problems among care recipients, including: "exacerbation of cognitive, functional, and neuropsychiatric problems in the care recipient."[49] Physical effects, social effects, financial effects, and psychological effects are other consequences associated with caregiver's burden. Specifically, dementia caregivers "have 46% more visits to the doctor, 71% more prescribed medications, higher diastolic blood pressure, higher noradrenalin levels, lower cell-mediated immunity, 63% higher mortality risk, and poorer self-rated health," when compared with matched non-caregiver controls, according to this report.[50]

A large body of research literature shows that caregivers experience stress, burden, depression, and a variety of physical health changes in response to their caregiving role.[51] Dang and his colleagues provide a number of examples. They report that social effects are linked to the demands of caregiving. Caregivers often find they are forced to abandon leisure activities and spend less time with friends and family. As a consequence, caregivers may experience feelings of isolation or loneliness. Resentment may also occur as some caregivers start to feel overwhelmed by circumstances over which they have no control. This may, in turn, result in their harboring feelings of being cheated in some way. Other psychological effects may include a high incidence of depression, anxiety, and psychotropic drug use along with poor perceived health status and higher health-care utilization when compared to controls matched for age, gender, race, and marital status.[52]

Moreover, direct and indirect financial effects may pose an additional burden for caregivers. Dang et al. report that although indirect costs are difficult to keep track of, they may include such things as "the value of caregiving time, the caregiver's lost income, out-of-pocket expenses for formal caregiving services, and the caregiver's excess health costs. The demands of caregiving may eventually make it impossible for the caregiver to continue work."[53]

The Sandwich Generation
A popular term has been coined for adult children who provide caregiving for their senior parents; they have come to be known as the *sandwich generation*. This term is associated with the fact that younger caregivers often find themselves "sandwiched" between caregiving responsibilities associated with caring for children and caring for elderly parents. Statistics show that caregivers

"provide an average of 70 hours of care a week, and many are 'on-call' 24 hours a day, seven days a week, without relief." Furthermore, the average dementia patient lives from 2 to 20 years, and the average caregiving duration is about five years.[54] This group of baby boomers is not only responsible for their aging parents but also for their nuclear families as well. "With the youngest boomers nearing the age of 50, we expect the number of those assuming a caregiver role to rise steadily over the next decade," said Laurent Smith. This growth in the "sandwich generation" will be accompanied by increased opportunities to address their emotional concerns and needs, Smith concludes.[55]

Caregiving can be a full-time commitment that is made more complicated when the demands of work and family are factored into the equation. Under some circumstances the caregiver's life can become a difficult balancing act causing many members of the sandwich generation to feel stretched and emotionally drained. These feelings are especially difficult for those caregivers who remember their parents as vibrant and active people. If disregarded, the stress of caregiving can lead to burnout, damaging the caregiver's physical and mental health. That's why it is important for caregivers to take some time to care for themselves by actively attending to the emotional strain and the physical toll of taking care of others. Otherwise, compassion fatigue and caregivers' burden begin to have an impact on the caregiving relationship.

End of Chapter Exercises

Familial Caregiving and Care Receiving When Verbal Skills Are Limited

The case will focus on the interaction of the caregiver with the care recipient at the end stages of Alzheimer's disease.

Vignette: Mr. Jones who is 80 years old has been caring for his 75-year-old wife, who was diagnosed with Alzheimer's disease six years ago. The illness has progressed to the point at which she is in a vegetative state. They continue to live in their own home with the support of hospice. She is bedridden; she does not speak nor acknowledge the presence of her husband except for a slight eye reflex movement in response to his voice. When encouraged to seek respite by his family and friends, Mr. Jones replies, "I will not leave her bedside . . . the occasional movement of her eyes is enough for me to live on."

Case Study Analysis Questions
1. Define the nature of the problem.
2. Use specific details that provide sufficient background for analysis.
3. Evaluate the seriousness of the problem.
4. Determine the extent to which some kind of action is required immediately.
5. Identify two or more alternative solutions.
6. Describe a particular course of action and describe your rationale for selecting it.
7. Describe a plan to implement the action you selected.

Chapter Four – Theme Three: Holism and Equilibrium

Theme Summary

Theme 3: Caregiving influences the equilibrium of familial and non-familial social systems.

Emotional, psychological, and social influences in caregiving were expressed in both positive and negative terms for this theme. As noted in the comments, both familial and non-familial influences are important. Another common thread running through these comments was maintaining equilibrium. Caregiving involves a significant change in one's lifestyle. Such far reaching change in one aspect of the caregiver's life must be accompanied by adjustments in the other areas in order to achieve harmony.

Survey responses

Some participants reported varying degrees of frustration, anger, and confusion in relation to their caregiving responsibilities. One participant said, "Sometimes I did feel alone and trapped, but this was not a constant. Some days were not as bad as others. Some days, I feel very resentful and angry." Another reported, "I don't understand why my siblings stop caring." A different participant noted: "My sister and I had other siblings who did not pull their share of the care, but tended to be opinionated on whatever we did in terms of direct care."

On a more positive note, a different participant was encouraged by the support received from family and church members: "My brother helped for a while and several church members volunteered their support and time. It helped me a lot." Another participant described the way she compensated by relying on friends:

"I would invite my friends over more than usual because of caring for my mom. My mom enjoyed having people over; it was company for her as well as for me. I also was part of a hospice group, which allowed me to place my mom in the hospice home while I went out of town. They also provided home care three times a week for a couple of hours."

Relevant Academic Literature

Relying on social systems such as friends, family members, community services, and support groups emerged as an effective influence in the well-being of caregivers. One study says:

"Some caregivers describe the caregiving experience as enriching their life and claim a high level of satisfaction with the caregiving role. They experience an improved quality of interpersonal relationships, an increased sense of competency in the role, and have a feeling of efficacy from dealing with problems. Positive caregiving produces a delay in institutionalization of the care recipient."[56]

Sanders has noted that in one research study, the caregivers indicated that support groups were "important for not only the support that they provided, but also the honesty of the group members."[57] Additionally, some caregivers believed that participating in support groups represented a way to 'give back' to other caregivers through "advice, recommendations, and serving as an emotional presence."[58] A similar study cited Kramer, who reported that: "Caregiving for an older family member can be a satisfying and rewarding experience despite the possible stress of managing one's whole life."[59]

Marks, Lambert, and Choi have identified a number of individual and personal rewards and benefits associated with caregiving.[60] They report that caregiving offers an opportunity to adult children to repay a parent for what they describe as many years of loving care. Caregivers in this situation also tend to experience personal gratification from doing a job well. The authors further note that "Sometimes, just being with the older person can be rewarding." On a different note, Marks et al. also indicate that caregiving tends to coincide with the developmental demands of middle age. In this regard, these authors report that issues "from the caregiver's adolescence or childhood may arise through intentional reflection or abruptly surface from deep recesses of the unconscious mind. Whether the act of caregiving induces an attentive mindfulness … or abrupt catharsis, caring for a parent or grandparent frequently fosters occasions to *resolve past hurts and conflicts.*"[61] Other benefits of caregiving, according to these authors, include developing strength and aging readiness. In fact these authors go on to suggest that "the complexities of caregiving can make caregivers' lives chaotic and increase their vulnerability to stress-related illness; however, many caregivers experience growth through the chaos."[62] They conclude that:

It is not unusual for caregivers of older family members to have a higher level of personal comfort as they approach their own maturity. This is primarily because they have shed a certain amount of their naiveté about the aging process; now less pessimistic, they are able to recognize a range of qualities that accompany aging in themselves and others. Not only that, they tend to understand that "deriving enjoyment from an older family member requires conscious presence and awareness of the person-who-is-there."[63]

Implications for Caregivers

Caregivers attend to all aspects of the caregiving relationship.

Effective Communication: When Words Are Not Enough

To maintain the quality of the relationship between caregiver and care recipient, it is imperative that the lines of communication remain open. Detection of early signs of dementia is a very important task for the family caregiver and is at the basis of a good foundation for productive communication.[64] The speech of the Alzheimer's patient may run the course of going from coherent to sporadic moments of clarity to "word salad" and eventually, the care recipient may become mute. As memory fades and speech declines, alternative mechanisms of communication must be identified. The senses also have an influence on the manner in which people communicate. If the care recipient is experiencing low vision, the use of seeing the face of the caregiver and perhaps watching the lips for word cues will be greatly diminished. With age-related hearing loss, the coupling of seeing and hearing to enhance communication will be impaired. Of course, gentle touching based on the preference of the care recipient can enhance the communication process. Smelling and tasting can also be used carefully to enhance communication when appropriate. Keeping the living environment consistent, uncluttered, and simple can contribute to productive communication. Caregivers need to be aware that catastrophic events such as tornados, hurricanes, and earthquakes by nature will contribute the difficulties in communication. It is wise to plan ahead for such periods.

Impact of Dementia on Communication
Communication abilities of people with Alzheimer's are affected differently during the early, middle, and late stages of the disease.[65] Stages are based on documented common patterns of symptom progression of Alzheimer's disease. Symptoms and progress vary from person to person. Although the duration of the disease can vary from three to 20 years, people with Alzheimer's die an average of four to six years after diagnosis.[66]

Psychological Impact
Several psychological issues are of significant concern for the recipients of care. These issues are depression, hopelessness, helplessness, and low-esteem. Depression, as described earlier, is frequently an intrapersonal response to chronic physical illness. Hopelessness can be defined as having no expectation of success and no anticipation of resolution or a positive outcome. Hopelessness is closely related to depression.[67]

Hopelessness if not addressed by the caregiver, can spark the beginning phases of resignation and "giving up" on the part of the care recipient. Learned helplessness, a related concept, can be defined as a behavioral state and personality trait of a person who believes that he or she is ineffectual, his or her responses are futile, and control over reinforcers in the environment has been lost. For the geriatric care recipient, learned helplessness could refer to a condition in which a person attempts to establish and maintain contact with another by adopting an over-dependent, powerless stance.[68]

Self-esteem reflects an individual's overall evaluation or appraisal of his or her own worth. Level and quality of self-esteem are distinct aspects of the concept. One can exhibit high but fragile self-esteem (i.e. narcissism) or low but stable self-esteem (i.e. humility). Historically, research investigators who have examined the quality of self-esteem have focused on constancy over time (stability), independence of meeting particular conditions (non-contingency) and in terms of ingrained nature on a basic psychological level (implicitness).[69]

It is important to remember that patients with dementia need to be "accepted, to be given worth and honor, to be befriended and to be listened to, to be placed within a wider context of peace and security, of beauty and love."[70] These patients are especially vulnerable and may be lonely and bewildered. Using interventions such as Reminiscence Therapy can be effective as a way to counteract depression.

Reminiscence Therapy
Reminiscence Therapy (RT) involves the discussion of past activities, events, and experiences with another person or group of people, usually with the aid of tangible prompts such as photographs, household and other familiar items from the past, music and archive sound recordings.[71] Reminiscence groups typically involve group meetings in which participants are encouraged to talk about past events at least once a week. Life review typically involves individual sessions, in which the person is guided chronologically through life experiences and encouraged to evaluate them. At the conclusion of these sessions, the care recipient may produce a life story book. Family caregivers are increasingly involved in reminiscence therapy. Reminiscence therapy is one of the most popular psychosocial interventions in dementia care, and is highly rated by staff and participants. There is some evidence to suggest it is effective in improving mood in older people without dementia. Its effects on mood, cognition, and well-being in dementia are less well understood.

Reminiscence therapy involves the process of remembering the past either spontaneously or guided by a therapist, with or without props. It is a technique frequently used to support older people. This form of therapeutic intervention respects the life and experiences of the individual and often helps the patient to maintain good mental health. It relies primarily on remote memory functions, the last functions to be eroded as we age. Reminiscence can occur in one-to-one or group format. The group often determines the content of a particular session, and the leaders of the group use their skills in ensuring that all participants are respected and have their opportunity to take part. The therapist may use music, photographs, replica documents, drama, and sensory gardens to stimulate discussion for the participants. Reminiscence therapy is a useful tool in supporting very frail and confused people to integrate into new living arrangements while respecting them and their life history.

Reminiscence therapy is an independent nursing intervention that may be helpful in maintaining or improving self-esteem and life satisfaction for the elderly, but the effects of reminiscence therapy are difficult to measure.[72] Lin et al. shed some understanding of reminiscence as a nursing therapeutic in a recent research article. This article reviewed the developmental history and theoretical basis of reminiscence and evaluated the empirical evidence concerning the use and effectiveness of reminiscence in the elderly. A lack of consistent research findings resulted from selecting different therapeutic goals, different types of reminiscence, different dependent measures, different data collection tools, different sample populations, and small sample size. Future nursing research should redefine the concept and attempt to standardize the measurement of reminiscence and then forge ahead using rigorous research designs to develop a body of knowledge regarding reminiscence.[73]

Reminiscence Literature
The following articles provide a good overview of the concept of reminiscence therapy. Interest in psychiatric nursing as a practice area is associated with positive undergraduate clinical experiences that include staff acceptance, diverse learning opportunities, direct involvement with care recipients, and community placements, according to Perese, Simon, and Riley. [74] Essential student preparedness includes attitudes affirmative of patient recovery; assessment, communication, teaching, and medication administration and monitoring skills; and a toolkit of nursing interventions such as group facilitation and reminiscence therapy. In an innovative intervention, students in a geriatric psychiatric community setting developed and facilitated a support group with reminiscence-based activities to reduce social isolation. Care recipients increased social interactions, and students gained awareness of older adults' interests and self-identities, as well as confidence in providing care. [75]

Chao, Chen, Liu, and Clark[76] designed a study to develop an understanding of the process of reminiscence and the roles played by nurses in fostering reminiscence as a therapeutic intervention. Reminiscence therapy has been considered an effective nursing strategy for improving quality of life and preventing depression in nursing home settings. Until recently, however, there has been little attention to understanding the dynamics of reminiscence therapy and the interaction between a nurse and an older client during reminiscence. A qualitative research design employing participant observation and content analysis of recorded reminiscence therapy sessions was used in this study. Participant observation was used to explore the process of individual reminiscence therapy and identify nursing roles in the process generated. Ten nursing home residents participated and data were collected over two months

through interviews and observation. Content analysis was used to identify emerging themes. Reminiscence occurred in four stages: entree, immersion, withdrawal, and closure. Stimuli related to participants' past
lives were helpful for initiating reminiscence. Nursing roles in each stage were identified. A tentative model of the process of reminiscence was derived from study findings.

Complementary therapies (CTs) are gaining popularity in the general population, including cancer patients, according to Kozachik, Wyatt, Given, and Given.[77] Yet, little is known about characteristics differentiating the use of one versus more CTs, about the patterns and persistence of CT use over time, or about the characteristics of cancer patients and their family caregivers who elect to participate in a study involving the use of CTs. The focus of this quasi-experimental study was to offer an eight-week, five-contact, nurse-delivered intervention involving guided imagery, reflexology, and reminiscence therapy to cancer patients undergoing chemotherapy and their family caregivers. Participants were allowed to elect to use none or any combination of CTs. Twenty-seven percent of eligible patients signed consent forms and agreed to participate. The typical participant was Caucasian, married, and had at least a high school education. Higher levels of education predicted use of more than one CT among cancer patients; there were no significant predictors for caregivers. Female patients were more likely to complete the CT protocol than their male counterparts, but there were no associations between CT protocol completion and caregiver demographics. Patients and family caregivers who elected to use more than one CT did not consistently implement their CTs. Participants who elected to use only one CT were more consistently performing their CT over time, suggesting that this lower level of CT use may be easier to integrate into their lives during cancer treatment.

The need to provide quality mental health care for elders in nursing home settings has been a critical issue, as the aging population grows rapidly and institutional care becomes a necessity for some elders.[78] The purpose of this quasi-experimental study was to describe the effect of participation in reminiscence group therapy on older nursing home residents' depression, self-esteem, and life satisfaction. Purposive sampling was used to recruit participants who met the study criteria. Residents of one ward were assigned to the reminiscence therapy group intervention, while residents of the other ward served as controls. Nine weekly one-hour sessions were designed to elicit reminiscence as group therapy for 12 elders in the experimental group. Another 12 elders were recruited for a control group matched to experimental subjects on relevant criteria. Depression, self-esteem, and life satisfaction were measured one week before and after the therapy. Results indicated that group reminiscence therapy significantly improved self-esteem, although effects on depression and life satisfaction were not significant. Reminiscence groups could enhance elders' social interaction with one another in nursing home settings and become support groups for participants. The model created here can serve as a reference for future application in institutional care.

Two reviewers independently extracted data and assessed trial quality. Five trials are included in the review, but only four trials with a total of 144 participants had extractable data. The results were statistically significant for cognition (at follow-up), mood (at follow-up) and on a measure of general behavioral function (at the end of the intervention period). The improvement on cognition was evident in comparison with both no treatment and social contact control conditions. Caregiver strain showed a significant decrease for caregivers participating in groups with their relative with dementia, and staff knowledge of group members' backgrounds improved significantly. No harmful effects were identified on the outcome measures reported.[79]

The purpose of a study conducted by Jones was to determine the effects of a three-week, six-session Nursing Interventions Classification (NIC) reminiscence intervention on the level of depression among elderly women residing in one assisted-living long-term care facility using a pre-test--post-test, quasi-experimental design.[80] A convenience sample of 30 women (M = 81.7 years) participated in the study. Participants were randomly assigned to one of two groups, an experimental group that received the NIC reminiscence intervention and a comparison group that received the customary reminiscence intervention used within the assisted living long-term care facility. Depression was measured using the Geriatric Depression Scale. Pre-test geriatric depression scores revealed the initial levels of depression were similar for participants in both the experimental and control groups. Post-test geriatric depression scores indicated those participating in the NIC reminiscence group had significantly lower depression scores compared to those participating in the facility's customary reminiscence group. The findings of this study suggest that a nurse-initiated intervention, NIC reminiscence therapy, was an effective treatment in reducing symptoms of depression among elderly women.

Holistic Approaches for Care Recipients
A growing number of health care professionals believe that the care of dementia and Alzheimer's patients must be holistic. That is, their needs must be addressed "from not only a physical perspective but from mental, psychosocial and spiritual perspectives as well."[81] One article reminds us that:

Anandarajah and Hight remind us about the multidimensional aspect of the human experience, of which spirituality is an important component. It is difficult, if not impossible, to fully measure each dimension using the scientific method. At the same time, however, convincing evidence is appearing in the medical literature to support the importance of spirituality in the practice of medicine. These researchers note that "It will take many more years of study to understand exactly which aspects of spirituality hold the most benefit for health and well-being." [82] This author agrees with their assessment that many of the world's great wisdom traditions have noted that important aspects of the spiritual link to wellness may not be measureable. They encompass things like having a sense of connection and inner strength; possessing comfort, love, and peace derived from meaningful relationships with self, others, and nature; and acknowledging and embracing transcendence.[82]

Background and Relevance of Holism
A major premise of this book is that attending to the holistic needs of caregivers can have an impact on their overall quality of life and can carry over into the quality of care for their loved ones. There has been increased interest in holistic approaches to mental health in recent years. A major holism movement occurred in the early 20th century with the appearance of Gestalt psychology and the

psychology of perception. Gestalt psychology had an influence on Gestalt Therapy as conceptualized by Fritz Perls. At the basis of Perls' therapy was gestalt theory which had a significant influence on the "phenomenology of perception."[83]

In teleological psychology, the pioneer psychologist Alfred Adler believed that the individual was an integrated whole expressed through a self-consistent unity of thinking, feeling, and action. Further, as a social member of the larger whole of mankind, the need must exist to take an interest in the welfare of others, as well as a respect for nature. These concepts are at the heart of Adler's philosophy of living and the principles of psychotherapy.[84] Moreover, some counselors and researchers have begun to inquire into the spiritual aspects of depression, for example. Diagnostic criteria for mental disorders are essentially descriptions of symptoms which fall into several categories. In major depressive disorders, affective or mood symptoms include depressed mood and feelings of worthlessness or guilt. Behavioral symptoms include social withdrawal and agitation. Cognitive symptoms or problems in thinking include difficulty with concentration or making decisions. Finally, somatic or physical symptoms include insomnia or sleeping too much.[85]

Theorists have explored the role of spirituality in human growth and actualization but also have questioned the impact of the lack of a spiritual perspective on mental health in general. Seligman[86] has linked increased feelings of helplessness and hopelessness to the narcissism of our time. Contrary to the growing levels of depression in the larger society, Seligman observed the low, stable levels of depression among the spiritual community of the Amish in Pennsylvania. These theorists have advanced strong arguments for the importance of spirituality to mental health. Not only have they argued for the valid and vital role of spirituality in human growth and actualization, but they also have suggested that a link exists between a lack of spirituality and lower levels of mental health, including increased feelings of hopelessness, meaninglessness, and depression.

As noted earlier in this discussion, some counselors view spirituality as transcendence or the awareness of and appreciation for the vastness of the universe. The term also encompasses recognition of a dimension "beyond the natural and rational,"[87] as well as an acceptance of its mystery and an element of faith.[88] Transcendence can include an awareness of or belief in a force greater than oneself, whether this be God, an infinite being or beings, or a cosmic force.[89]

Maintaining Equilibrium
In the 1990s Robert Restak wrote a book called *The Brain Has a Mind of Its Own*.[90] His text described the relationship between the mind and the brain in terms of neurology or the study of the brain and its disorders. His argument was built on recent technology including imaging techniques and genetic studies showing that "many emotional illnesses are heredity and associated with physical alterations in the genome."[91] He used the electroencephalogram as an example of technology that could measure the brain's electrical activity to reveal things like epilepsy. In one of his essays Restak alludes to the 17th century philosopher Rene Descartes who conjectured that the human body is a machine involving functions that can be explained by mathematical laws of physics. Restak concedes, however, that at the same time, technology is incapable of revealing

the whole picture. As supported by the principles of quantum physics, the conclusions we reach based on our observations depend to a large extent on our perspective. In other words, a dualism is at work. Restak reports:

"When I listen to my patients tell me about a frightening vision or hallucination – something far removed from everyday experience – I'm encountering the world of mind. But if I record my patient's brain waves during hallucination and detect an epileptic seizure within the temporal lobe, I've shifted my focus ... from one aspect of reality to another."[92]

Beverly Engel also has focused her attention on the mind, its connection with the body, and the need for emotional awareness. She tells us that:

"Your body is your best barometer to tell you which emotion you are feeling at any given time. Emotions involve body changes, such as fluctuations in heart rate and skin temperature and the tensing or relaxing of muscles. The most important changes are in the facial muscles. Researchers now think that changes in these muscles play an important role in actually causing emotions."[93]

She describes how our body language can give clues to our emotional states and indicates that frowning, drooping eyes, and slumped posture, for example, can all be indicators of sadness, one of our primary emotions. Other indicators might be "moist eyes or tears, whimpering, crying, feeling as if you can't stop crying; or feeling that if you ever start crying you will never stop.[94] Others have observed similar connections. Today a growing number of medical professionals are acknowledging a correlation between mind and body processes. Moreover, the concepts of holism are being incorporated to a greater extent in the curricula for medical professionals.

Andrew Weil, a doctor of osteopathic medicine and bestselling author, recognizes the power of what he considers to be the untapped potential of mind/body healing. In his book *Spontaneous Healing* he provides anecdotal evidence of psychosomatic (mind/body) remission of serious diseases, including cancer.[95] Weil comments on the correlation between healing in people with chronic illness and a transcendent entity:

"The most common correlation I observe between mind and healing in people with chronic illness is total acceptance of the circumstances of one's life, including illness. This change allows profound internal relaxation, so that people need no longer feel compelled to maintain a defensive stance toward life. Often, it occurs as part of a spiritual awakening and submission to a higher power."[96]

How are emotions and physical symptoms related to the spirit? As rational beings, humans have free will or the ability to select from infinite choices. Our mental, physical, and spiritual "faculties" work in tandem to govern our decisions. As we acquire information we develop habits of mind, which influence our habits of behavior and our sense of spiritual well-being. Just as the body can indicate emotional distress, our emotions can likewise give us clues to the sources of our spiritual unrest. This unrest manifests in a persistent nudging sensation that begs our attention and urges us to explore and resolve the tension. Only then can we find resolution and peace. Thus, the relationship among mind, body, and spirit is a holistic one, which requires equilibrium among all components.

End of Chapter Exercise

This case will focus on the caregiver's need to understand the goals of reminiscence therapy groups.

Vignette: Mrs. Adams, who resides in a skilled nursing care facility, was asked by staff to participate in ongoing reminiscence therapy groups. Until this point, Mrs. Adams spent her days in her wheelchair in the patient sittings room, communicating only when spoken too by staff and exhibiting a "flat" expressionless affect. She rarely responded to other residents of the nursing care facility. After one month of participating in the reminiscence group, Mrs. Adams was able to make connections with other patients and share happy, as well as, sad memories of her life with others. One day, her 45-year-old adult daughter approached the staff leader of the reminiscence group to complain about a sad memory which had caused her mother to cry. The daughter stated that she did not mind her mother reminiscing about happy periods in her life but felt that when her mother reminisced about the more emotion laden sad period in her life she might "lose control of herself." The daughter requested that her mother no longer participate in the reminiscence therapy groups because they might "upset her."

Case Study Analysis Questions

1. Define the nature of the problem.
2. Use specific details that provide sufficient background for analysis.
3. Evaluate the seriousness of the problem.
4. Determine the extent to which some kind of action is required immediately.
5. Identify two or more alternative solutions.
6. Describe a particular course of action and describe your rationale for selecting it.
7. Describe a plan to implement the action you selected.

Chapter Five –
Theme Four: Spiritual Discipline

Theme Summary

Theme 4: Spiritual discipline can ease the strain of caregiving.

Spiritual support can come from many sources including family, friends, health care providers, and clergy. Spiritual care activities can be varied and often include prayer, religious ritual, or services. Spiritual well-being is also associated with other forms of self-care, which can "take the form of reconnecting with family and friends, time alone (for quiet contemplation, playing a sport, recreational reading, nature watching, etc.), community service or religious practice."[97]

Survey Responses

Spiritual well-being emerged as an important theme among participants. Many of their comments related to establishing balance as a common component necessary for them to maintain an overall level of well-being.[98] When asked to identify specific activities that were most effective in helping them care for their own spiritual needs participants responded with the following.

- *"Taking a few minutes alone when I can just sit and breathe."*

- *"Bible Study, Sunday School, Personal devotional time."*

- *"I engage in a rigorous spiritual discipline each morning that includes prayer, scripture reading, and critical reflection along with journaling."*

- *"Attending or viewing positive religious services on television."*

- *"Daily prayer and not taking each moment so seriously."*

- *"Bible reading, prayer, Bible class and fellowship with Christian friends."*

- *"Going to Church, prayer for patience, knowing that God is willing and able to stick with you."*

- *"Disciple classes."* (2 participants)

- *"I pray, do devotionals, attend church, and listen to religious music."*

- *"Praying, talking to my mom, going out with friends for conversations and support."*

- *"Thinking positively."*

- *"Active church involvement."*

Many of these activities are religious in nature; others are not. Spirituality is an important aspect of the human experience. Many of the caregivers who responded to the survey felt that their spiritual faith enhanced their overall well-being. This helped them to avoid spiritual distress and spiritual crisis, which occur "when individuals are unable to find sources of meaning, hope, love, peace, comfort, strength, and connection in life or when conflict occurs between their beliefs and what is happening in their life."[99] The Mayo Foundation reminds us that expressions of spirituality can involve a range of activities, including those associated with religious traditions, such as prayer and attending church services. In fact, religious involvement and spirituality overlap in a number of ways. Spirituality doesn't always have to be connected to a specific belief or form of worship. On the contrary; quite often and for many people, "spirituality is simply a search for meaning, values and purpose in life. At times spirituality is expressed through emotional forms such as music, meditation, or art. Some people satisfy their spiritual yearnings by seeking harmony with nature and the universe."[100]

Relevant Academic Literature

Spiritual well-being is defined as "sense of peace and contentment stemming from an individual's relationship with the spiritual aspects of life." Some sources report that "All people have spiritual selves that depend on emotions, feelings, and intellectual ability. This self integrates other aspects of life."[101] Most research on caregivers' burden concentrates on medical and psychosocial well-being. However, spiritual needs of caregivers are now receiving greater attention. A growing body of research indicates that spirituality plays a beneficial role in the practice of medicine[102] and that patients as well as caregivers believe that spirituality plays an important role in their lives. These studies indicate that there is a positive correlation between a patient's spirituality or religious commitment and health outcomes.

Recent research studies support this view. One research study, conducted by Sanders et al., concludes that spiritual distress can have an adverse effect on mental and physical health. Participants in this study made it clear that "without faith in God, their ability to persevere as a caregiver would have been compromised."[103] For many caregivers, faith engenders hope, which according to Dunne, is transcendent in nature and consists of a kind of knowledge "because it anticipates a beyond, a resolution of all chaos, and an ultimate meaning to the universe whatever our personal role in it."[104] This same study also noted that caregivers struggled with "managing their own spiritual needs and knowing how to help a loved one in spiritual distress."

In a different research study, Scott and his colleagues concluded that "spiritual care recognizes the relationship between illness and the spiritual domain, and acknowledges the possibility of a search for meaning in the big questions of life and death."[105] Having a systematic set of religious beliefs is important for some people. According to Scott et al.:

"[People] who claimed to have no religious belief acknowledged that they might pray in times of particular adversity. Our data suggest that people utilize a wide range of coping strategies. Spiritual needs were expressed in terms of the need to maintain a sense of self and self-worth, to have a useful role in life, retaining an active role with family and friends."[106]

Implications for Caregivers

Spirituality and Well-Being

Although more is known about caring for the mental and physical needs of Alzheimer's patients, issues of the spirit have been shown to be an important component of any care plan. The Mayo Medical Foundation reminds us that for Alzheimer's care recipients "spirituality, faith and religious rituals can be important for overall well-being. If you're a caregiver for someone with Alzheimer's disease, helping your loved one continue to observe his or her faith can be beneficial and rewarding for both of you."[107] Not only that; religious commitment was helpful in the prevention of illness (including depression, substance abuse, and physical illness) in coping with illness and in recovery from illness.[108]

Research studies highlight the importance of spiritual well-being for Alzheimer's patients along with their social, emotional, and psychological health, says Rev. Dr. Janet Aldrich, a chaplain in a suburban Chicago residential care facility for the elderly. She has noted that during dementia, the care recipient's need for spiritual connection and recognition of self do not diminish. "In fact, as all relational functions fail, the religious function is the last to be destroyed. Memory impaired persons still have emotions, imagination, will, and moral awareness far into the disease process of dementia."[109] Aldrich further asserts that although one pathway to creating a sense of spiritual relations and supporting the care recipient's personal sense of spiritual self can be found through religion, "religious needs and systems are not universal."[110]

Spirituality versus Religion
Spirituality takes many forms. While many people use the words *spirituality* and *religion* interchangeably, these terms are very different. Spirituality can be defined as a complex and multidimensional part of the human experience, a person's inner belief system. It helps individuals to search for the meaning and purpose of life, and it helps them experience hope, love, inner peace, comfort, and support. Religion, on the other hand, refers to a belief system to which an individual adheres. Religion involves rituals, practices, and other external symbols of a belief system. Many people find spirituality through religion while others find spirituality through communing with nature, music, the arts, quest for scientific truth, or a set of values and principles. Not everyone is religious; nor is religion a requirement for spirituality.

Spiritual assessment represents a way to help determine the extent to which a person's spirituality or religion may impact upon his or her well-being overall. Within a spiritual assessment, it is important to determine if a care recipient has a religious affiliation; however, that is not the sole purpose of the assessment. A person may not practice religion, but may still have spiritual needs that should be met. Any assessment process should identify these spiritual needs, in whatever form they take.[111]

Fortifying the linkage between the medical and the spiritual may involve systematic spiritual assessment as a practical way to begin incorporating spirituality into medical practice. Spiritual assessment is the process by which health care providers can identify a patient's spiritual needs pertaining to medical care.[112] According to Dang et al., those responsible for providing care to dementia recipients should be assessed routinely for their physical, emotional, and mental well-being. Assessment might include raising caregivers' awareness of depression and behavioral issues, and could increase caregivers' skill in dealing with the overall needs of the care recipient. All of this is done in an effort to avert "burn out," which can "open the door to potential instances of elder abuse and neglect."[113]

Spiritual Needs of Care Recipients
In "Through a Glass Darkly: A Dialogue between Dementia and Faith," Malcolm Goldsmith sheds additional light on spiritual needs of people with dementia:

"To be accepted, to be given worth and honor, to be befriended and to be listened to, to be placed within a wider context of peace and security, of beauty and love. They are the needs of all who are human, but with an extra dimension of sensitivity because people with dementia are especially vulnerable; they may be lonely and bewildered, they may be grieving and desperately trying to communicate, they are almost certainly frightened at some stage in their illness."[114]

Rev. Aldrich reinforces this point by drawing our attention to the specific spiritual dimensions of Alzheimer's patients. Regardless of their cognitive impairment, she notes, their "inward spirit which makes humans living beings continues with them until they actually die – not merely until they lose their cognitive faculties."[115] Aldrich further asserts that dementia alters all aspects of life – physical, mental, emotional, social, and religious – and distorts these aspects in unpredictable and confusing ways. As part of her work as chaplain in a residential retirement community, Rev. Aldrich has focused on residents with dementia and has implemented a radio program entitled "Worship for All God's Children." Through her observations and assessments, she has concluded that the care of dementia and Alzheimer's patients is best when it addresses a range of patients' needs.

Holistic Fitness for Caregivers

In order to provide optimum assistance to care recipients, caregivers need to maintain an overall level of personal fitness, and this fitness should be holistic in nature. The goal of holistic fitness, specifically, is to ensure that caregivers pay attention to their mental, physical, and spiritual needs as part of an integrated, balanced approach to wholeness. Whether we are talking about mental, physical, or spiritual fitness, a number of common components are necessary to maintain well-being. They are nourishment, exercise, respiration, and rest.

One common component to maintaining fitness is nourishment. Mental nourishment involves life-long stimulation of the mental faculties. Physical nourishment entails providing nutrients through diet or dietary supplements as well as adequate fluids necessary to sustain growth and development of the physical organism. Spiritual nourishment thrives on receptivity to the transcendent aspects of one's being.

The concept of fitness further requires engaging in exercise on a regular basis. Such exercise pertains equally to the mind, body, and spirit. For example, the mind is stretched by resolving cognitive dissonance, thinking critically, and visualizing. The body receives exercise through physical activity that is planned, structured, and repetitive for the purpose of conditioning the body. Physical exercise also improves health and prolongs life. The spirit engages in exercise through reading, reflecting, and meditating.

Respiration is another aspect of holistic fitness. To respire is to inhale or exhale. The mind respires through processing information as it assimilates or accommodates new ideas. Mental respiration also occurs through release of emotional tension. In a physical sense, the body breathes in order to facilitate metabolism during and after exertion. Spiritual respiration involves inhaling deeply of the spiritual breath of life and exhaling spiritual tension and anxiety.

Rest is equally as important. It facilitates recovery and restoration, which are components necessary to help the living system to thrive. Recovery and restoration might be accomplished through recreation or down time, as the mind, body, and spirit are replenished through sleep, play, amusement, or relaxation.

Each component – mind, body, and spirit – has its distinct indicators of fitness, yet at the same time all components are linked in complex ways. Because of these linkages, balance among all of the components is critical. Tranquility and peacefulness may be the byproducts of deliberate attempts to achieve holistic equilibrium as part of a plan for personal renewal. Renewal, restoration, and freedom from stress are likely to result in all three dimensions.

End of Chapter Exercises

Informal Caregiving and Care Receiving with Members of the Social Network

The case will focus on caregiving by a church member group.

Vignette: Sadie has been a member of a women's mission circle at her church for the last 20 years. She has no living biological relatives. However, she refers to the 12 ladies who comprise her mission circle as family members. Her peers have noticed that she is very forgetful, frequently asking them the same questions over and over again. She recently experienced a small fire in her home because she forgot to turn the oven and the stove-top off before living the house for a six-hour outing.

Case Study Analysis Questions

1. Define the nature of the problem.
2. Use specific details that provide sufficient background for analysis.
3. Evaluate the seriousness of the problem.
4. Determine the extent to which some kind of action is required immediately.
5. Identify two or more alternative solutions.
6. Describe a particular course of action and describe your rationale for selecting it.
7. Describe a plan to implement the action you selected.

Chapter Six – Theme Five: Shared Wisdom

Theme Summary

Theme 5: Seasoned caregivers have caregiving wisdom to share with others. Don't try to go it alone.

This conclusion emerges from a number of comments made by survey participants: "Get help from professional caregivers, spiritual advisors, and legal advisors. Understand that regardless of your personal relationship to and with the recipient you cannot meet all their and your needs alone. You need help," said one participant. Another participant summed it up: "Be strong; your strength is needed by the recipient as well as yourself."

Survey Results

One of the items on the survey asked caregivers: What advice do you have for people who are just now becoming caregivers? Suggestions varied. Most of the comments indicated that caregivers should seek help and advice from other people, to the extent possible. For example, one participant suggested that new caregivers should:

"Talk to the entire family to put a schedule together. When you begin to care for someone and do a good job, other family members think you are doing a great job and they do not need to assist other than infrequent visits. Burn out can occur very fast."

Another caregiver said:

"Push! Push everyone to work their hardest for you. Make them help you when you do not get the answers that you think you should. Don't just agree to what you are told; fight for what you think should be."

A different participant advised new caregivers to:

"Know that it can be very difficult without some assistance. And do not feel bad if some days you feel angry, because it's a normal reaction."

Having a support system in place was another suggestion:

"Maintain a balance as it relates to the time spent with your loved one and yourself. Have someone to whom you can vent! Have a support system (someone who can pick up the slack when you cannot do everything)."

Additional suggestions were provided by other participants. Their comments are provided on the following pages.

Acquire information needed to support responsible decision making. One of the participants commented: "Find out about the signs and symptoms of [the disease] as soon as possible. Check on your loved one often. Get to know his/her likes and dislikes so that when the cognitive functions begin to wane you might have other means of communicating with your loved one." A different participant said: "Make sure you are cognizant of the physical and emotional needs of the person you are providing care for. Seek out as many resources as you can to assist with caregiving. Also, develop a support system for yourself. Often caring for an elderly person is more taxing than caring for an infant...you have to take care of yourself in the process."

Use acquired information for advocacy. One of the participants suggested: "Be an advocate for your loved one – No one else will! Do not rely on the good will of the healthcare system – you'll likely be disappointed and in some cases outraged. Be spiritually anchored in faith. You may not get (feel) appreciation from other family members, but knowing that you've done all you could provides an incredible sense of peace and accomplishment."

Become familiar with the overall impact of the disease. One participant noted that new caregivers should: "Understand the amount of time that must be provided. Understand that it is o.k. to get away and let someone else care for your loved one. Understand that it is o.k. to be upset at the situation and sometimes not want to do it (I felt this way... but at no time did I give up). Get help from all available resources (government, family, church, and friends). Develop a relationship with your loved one's medical staff and make them explain everything. Be willing to ask questions until you are satisfied with the responses."

Heed practical advice. "Make sure you have lots of love to give, patience and time," said one participant. "Take care of yourself first!" said another. One of the participants summed it all up by saying: "Be prepared to deal with the best & worst of your family & be prepared to go it alone – [you] may not get much help or support from others."

Have a strong support system in place. One of the participants said that new caregivers should:

"Try to involve all your siblings and other family members. If you have a church home now is the time you really need their support; don't be afraid to ask. People can't read your mind; you have to let them know you need help and prayer. If your situation is headed towards a terminal

illness find a hospice group near your home; they provide several services during and after your loved one's illness. They even provide group sessions to help you express what you are going through."

Get some spiritual support. This was the suggestion of another participant. Along these same lines, information coupled with support was recommended by one of the participants. She advised new caregivers to: "Learn as much about the disease as possible. They should find a support group and get help with coping as much as possible."

Relevant Academic Literature

Research suggests that caregivers benefit from knowing that other caregivers have similar feelings. Being part of a support group can help caregivers develop active coping strategies as they seek information and confront issues. A number of studies have associated these activities with a lower occurrence of caregiver depression, burden, burnout, and other negative feelings such as panic and inadequacy.[116] Caregiver support groups received mixed reviews in home hospice situations.

Redinbaugh and her associates note that while some caregivers who use home hospice report that they are in need of social support, not all forms of social support are helpful. In some cases simple forms of support are needed as reported by at least one caregiver who simply needed someone to talk to in order to be reassured. With a different caregiver, the social support extended was perceived as burdensome. In this case, the caregiver simply wanted to be alone and sit quietly somewhere away from the hustle and bustle. He reported that: "people [kept] coming and going all the time and [I] didn't get any time alone."[117] Redinbaugh et al. conclude that psychological distress is not related directly to the number and quality of social resources available. Provision of practical, tangible assistance from other people enhanced both the overall physical and psychological health of the caregiver. Moreover, problem-solving strategies appeared to be important as a critical aspect of caregiver support groups.

Social support in conjunction with use of coping strategies enhanced adjustment among family caregivers of cancer patients, according to Redinbauth et al. Some of the caregivers used problem-focused coping mechanisms and tended to believe in the efficacy of their own approaches; these caregivers reported lower levels of strain than caregivers who used a different approach. In comparison, those caregivers who incorporated behaviors such as avoidance, passivity, self-blame, and resignation experienced greater levels of strain. The researchers acknowledge that relationships between caregiver stressor and caregiver strain should be studied in greater depth among patients with cancer. [118]

Many existing studies agree that support for caregivers should include education, practical counseling about common caregiving stresses, and referral to community resources.[119] One researcher reports that:

"Although not all interventions are helpful, there is strong agreement that improving caregiver knowledge about dementia, the caregiving role, and resources does benefit caregivers, a benefit that can be further extended by a multipronged approach targeting problem-solving skills, the care recipient's behavior, and the caregiver's own emotional response to caregiving."[120]

Implications for Caregivers

Questions and Answers on Keeping the Faith

How can deeply embedded information help patients?
The patient with Alzheimer's "may connect more easily with an old edition of a devotional book or hymnal than with the one currently used in your church or temple." Ask older relatives what the musical standards were when they were growing up. "The familiarity of verses and music, rendered much as they were in the past, may offer someone with Alzheimer's a comfort that goes beyond the words themselves." [121]

Is it possible for an Alzheimer's patient to attend religious services?
"Bringing someone with Alzheimer's to religious services isn't always easy because he or she may be disruptive. Some places of worship, however, have special rooms designed for parents to take noisy children. ... These areas could also be used for someone with Alzheimer's. If that's not an option, an early morning service may have fewer people in attendance." Other suggestions include: Going to church or temple between regular services and simply praying together. Getting families who have loved ones with Alzheimer's to gather at the same time every week to worship together. [122]

How can caregivers find relief?
Find a caregiver support group. These groups may provide a shoulder to cry on. Someone in the group may be able to take over the care of the person with Alzheimer's for a few hours. The group may simply provide a comforting presence. [123]

End of Chapter Exercises

Caregiving:
When the Care Receiver is Aggressive and Combative

The case will focus on caregiving in the home at the point that the behavior of the care recipient becomes difficult to manage and they must be placed in a long-term care facility.

Vignette: Mr. and Mrs. Adams promised each other early in their 60-year marriage that they would never place the other in a nursing home for any reason. Mr. Adams has started to leave the house wandering for hours at a time not telling Mrs. Adams where he is going. She has had to call the police on several occasions to help her find him. He is usually no more than three miles from the neighborhood in which they live. He has also started to become angry and belligerent for no apparent reason, accusing her of hiding things from him and plotting with her friends to get rid of him. Mrs. Adams loves her husband very much but has become fearful of him. Both her physical and her mental health have started to become impaired as a result of her daily stressful caregiving activities.

Case Study Analysis Questions
1. Define the nature of the problem.
2. Use specific details that provide sufficient background for analysis.
3. Evaluate the seriousness of the problem.
4. Determine the extent to which some kind of action is required immediately.
5. Identify two or more alternative solutions.
6. Describe a particular course of action and describe your rationale for selecting it.
7. Describe a plan to implement the action you selected.

Chapter Seven – Summary and Resources

Summary

In summary, even though the circumstances of each caregiver are slightly different, they share common themes with others functioning in that role. Chapter one provided the foundation for our discussion of caregivers' needs. It provided background, statistics, and introduced the study.

Chapter two revealed the value of reflective retrospection as a tool for caregivers to use. This skill does require pausing during the day-to-day, sometimes hectic, caregiver routine and momentarily stepping out of role to obtain a glimpse of objectivity about the caregiver-care recipient relationship.

Chapter three helped us to label strategies perhaps used for a lifetime as "positive coping strategies." This reframing process serves as an affirmation of functioning "OK" as a caregiver even when the outcomes are not "perfect."

Chapter four brought in a systems theory perspective in that, we are all bound together in time and space. Consequently, we need to be aware of our boundaries at all times and how our actions influence the actions of our care recipients and others with whom we come in contact.

Chapter five assisted us to get in touch with the spiritual dimension of our lives. We would not be complete nor function well without an in-depth awareness of this dimension.

Chapter six reinforced the need to share our wisdom and partake of the wisdom of others. You might say that this chapter is a take-off of the notion, "Why re-invent the wheel if you don't have to."

This book has defined, described, and analyzed issues concerning the needs of dementia caregivers, especially those suffering from Alzheimer's disease. Overall, it has attempted to provide advice, basic facts, and suggestions that caregivers might use to impact upon their own holistic well-being as well as that of care recipients. Coping with the ongoing stress of caregiving is difficult enough under the best of circumstances. We hope that the suggestions provided in this volume will make the job of caregiving less of a burden and transform it into a labor of love.

Resources and Agencies

The following links will point you to helpful agencies and other resources. We do not endorse one agency or resource provider over another. Nor do we promote any particular political, philosophical, religious, or social viewpoint or position. We have become aware of services provided here through referrals and word of mouth. We advise that you make your decisions carefully.

Agency	Contact Information
Administration on Aging	http://www.aoa.dhhs.gov/
Alzheimer's Association	http://www.alz.org/
American Hospice Foundation	http://www.americanhospice.org/
Alcoholics Anonymous	http://www.alcoholics-anonymous.org/
Alzheimer's Association 225 N. Michigan Ave., Ste. 1700 Chicago, IL 60601-7633 (800) 272-3900	http://alzheimers.org
Alzheimer's Disease Education and Referral (ADEAR) Center. P.O. Box 8250 Silver Spring, MD 20907-8250 Telephone: 800-438-4380 (toll-free)	http://www.nia.nih.gov/Alzheimers
Alzheimer's Foundation of America 322 Eighth Avenue, 7th Floor New York, NY 10001 866-232-8484 (toll-free)	http://www.alzfdn.org
American Association of	http://www.aarp.org

Agency	Contact Information
Retired Persons 800-424-3410	
American Medical Association (AMA) 800-621-8335	http://www.ama-assn.org/
Area Agencies on Aging (AAA)	http://www.aoa.dhhs.gov
Children of Aging Parents P.O. Box 167 Richboro, PA 18954-0167 800-227-7294 (toll-free)	http://www.caps4caregivers.org/
Eldercare Locator 800-677-1116 (toll-free)	http://www.eldercare.gov
Family Caregiver Alliance 180 Montgomery Street, Suite 1100 San Francisco, CA 94104 800-445-8106 (toll-free)	http://www.caregiver.org/
Family Caregiver Alliance National Center on Caregiving 180 Montgomery Street, Suite 1100 San Francisco, CA 94104 (415) 434-3388 or (800) 445-8106	http://www.caregiver.org/
National Alliance for Caregiving (NAC) 301-718-8444	http://www.caregiving.org
National Council on Aging 202-479-1200	http://www.ncoa.org
National Family Caregivers Association 10400 Connecticut Avenue, Suite 500 Kensington, MD 20895-3944 800-896-3650 (toll-free)	http://www.thefamilycaregiver.org

Agency	Contact Information
National Hospice and Palliative Care Organization 1700 Diagonal Road, Suite 625 Alexandria, VA 22314 800-658-8898 (toll-free)	http://www.nhpco.org/
National Institute on Aging Information Center 800-222-2225 (toll-free) 800-222-4225 (TTY/toll-free)	http://www.nia.nih.gov/ http://www.nia.nih.gov/Espanol
Online information center of the U.S. Administration on Aging 202-619-7501	http://www.healthfinder.gov/orgs/HR0060.htm
Simon Foundation for Continence P.O. Box 815 Wilmette, IL 60091 800-237-4666 (toll-free)	http://www.simonfoundation.org/
Well Spouse Association 63 West Main Street, Suite H Freehold, NJ 07788 800-838-0879 (toll-free)	http://www.wellspouse.org/

Hotlines

The following are helpful hotlines. We do not endorse one agency over another. Nor do we promote any particular political, philosophical, religious, or social viewpoint or position. We have become aware of the services provided here through referrals and word of mouth. We advise that you make your decisions carefully.

Agency Contact Information
Elder Abuse Hotline   800-279-0400
General Crisis Talk Line   800-999-9999

Assessing Spirituality

As Alzheimer's disease progresses, the care recipient may not be able to adequately communicate spiritual needs in a manner easily understood by others. In some cases, language may take on another form or disappear all together. Therefore, early assessments of spirituality are recommended.[124] Spiritual screening, spiritual history taking, and spiritual assessment constitute a continuum in the overall spiritual care of Alzheimer's patients.[125]

There are many levels of assessment. Spiritual screening, spiritual history taking, and spiritual assessment constitute a continuum in the overall spiritual care of Alzheimer's patients.[126] Spiritual screening attempts to identify and categorize basic spiritual needs that may be associated with spiritual risk, which in turn may contribute to poor health outcomes. Spiritual history taking entails collecting salient information used to formulate a comprehensive care plan. Spiritual assessment, on the other hand, comprises a full and objective investigation of a patient's spiritual life and history. While no single model of spiritual assessment has been identified as a standard, Paul Pruyser's model is used widely. Additional information about this model can be found in *The Minister as Diagnostician*. [127]

HOLISTIC FITNESS INVENTORY FOR CAREGIVERS

Dear Friend:

Are you a caregiver? If so, we need your help.

We are inviting you to participate in a confidential, non-scientific, informal survey to assess caregiver's burden. The survey will examine the opinions and behavior patterns of people who are or have been involved during the past 12 months in caregiving for aging adults.

Participation will consist of completing a demographic profile, answering three open-ended questions, and providing responses to short inventories. Completing these items should require no more than 20 minutes of your time.

Your involvement is voluntary and poses no risks to you as a participant. Your responses will be kept strictly confidential. Overall results from this survey will be used to raise awareness of the social, emotional, and spiritual needs of caregivers.

We sincerely appreciate your cooperation!

Best regards,

Lorrie C. Reed, PhD
Executive Director, Center Street Consulting

Part I: Demographic Information

1. When were you born?
    a. Before 1946
    b. Between 1946 and 1964
    c. Between 1965 and 1984
    d. Later than 1985

2. In what setting do you / did you provide most of your caregiving?
    a. Home
    b. Nursing home
    c. Hospital
    d. Hospice
    e. Other – Comment: (500 characters or less)

3. What was / is the nature of the care recipient's illness?
    a. Dementia
    b. Cancer
    c. Stroke
    d. Other

4. What is / was your relationship to the care recipient?

5. Are you currently providing care to this recipient?
    a. Yes
    b. No

6. For how long have you been / were you a caregiver?
    a. Less than 1 year
    b. 1 to 5 years
    c. More than 5 years

7. How much time do you / did you spend in giving care?
    a. Less than 6 hours a week
    b. 6 to 10 hours a week
    c. 11 to 20 hours a week
    d. More than 20 hours a week

8. What is your gender?
    a. Male
    b. Female

9. What is your race?
   a. Caucasian American
   b. African American
   c. Latino/a American
   d. Asian American
   e. Other

10. What is your marital status?
    a. Married
    b. Separated or divorced or widowed
    c. Single, never married
    d. Other

11. What is your employment status?
    a. Employed
    b. Retired
    c. Unemployed
    d. Other

12. What is your level of education?
    a. Did not complete high school
    b. Some college, but no degree
    c. Bachelor's degree
    d. Master's degree
    e. Beyond master's degree
    f. Other

13. Do you have children who are relying on your help in some way?
    a. Yes
    b. No

Part II: Holistic Fitness Inventory

14. Place a check mark in the space that indicates your degree of agreement with each statement. Answer each question as it applies to your situation within the past 12 months. Use the following scale: SD = Strongly Disagree, D = Disagree, A = Agree, SA = Strongly Agree.

	SD	D	A	SA
I exercise at least once a month.				
I consider myself to be a spiritual person.				
I do leisurely reading at least once a week.				
I work until I am exhausted on most days.				
I pray at least once a day.				
I find time for play at least once a week.				
Comment (500 characters or less)				

Part III: Open-Ended Items

15. Think about the time when you first became a caregiver, then respond to the following probe: "If I knew then what I know now, I would..." (1000 characters of less)

16. What specific activities are most effective in helping you care for your own spiritual needs?

17. What advice do you have for people who are just now becoming caregivers?

Part IVa: Subjective Caregiving Burden

18. Place a check mark in the space that indicates your degree of agreement with each statement. Answer each question as it applies to your situation within the past 12 months. Use the following scale: SD = Strongly Disagree, D = Disagree, A = Agree, SA = Strongly Agree.

	SD	D	A	SA
Your health has suffered because of the care you must give.				
You feel isolated and alone as the result of giving care.				
You have lost control of your life since having to give care.				
You are very tired as a result of giving care.				
You feel nervous or depressed when giving care.				
You feel trapped when giving care.				
You feel angry when you are around the relative who needs care.				
You feel you will be unable to give care much longer.				
You don't have enough money to care for your loved one.				
You feel resentful of other relatives who could help, but do not.				
Comment: (500 characters or less)				

Part IVb: Impact of Caregiving

19. Place a check mark in the space that indicates your degree of agreement with each statement. Answer each question as it applies to your situation within the past 12 months. Use the following scale: SD = Strongly Disagree, D = Disagree, A = Agree, SA = Strongly Agree.

	SD	D	A	SA
You wish you could just leave your caregiving to someone else.				
Your social life has suffered because you are giving care.				
You don't feel you have enough time for yourself.				
It's hard for you to plan things ahead of time because of caregiving.				
The patient's needs mostly determine how your days are spent.				
Your loved one asks for more help than is necessary.				
Your relationship with other family members is negatively affected.				
Giving care doesn't allow you as much privacy as you would like.				
You feel uncomfortable having friends over because of your loved one.				
Giving care has interfered with your use of space in your home.				
Comment (500 characters or less)				

Thank you for your cooperation!

TIPS FOR CAREGIVERS

TIPS FOR MAKING THE BEST OF THE SITUATION [128]

- Think about ways that caregiving has made you a stronger person.
- Think about why you have accepted this role and any positive aspects of caregiving.
- Think about the positive ways in which caregiving and the patient's illness have changed your relationship with the patient.
- Consider if caregiving has brought you closer to the patient and/or other relatives or friends.
- Make a list of positive aspects of your relationship with the patient, shared memories, and what the patient means to you. Look at the list whenever you find yourself getting upset about the situation.

TIPS FOR RELIEVING STRESS

Many of the stress busters provided here were suggested by the Montana State University Extension Service of the United States Department of Agriculture.[129] Other items come from the authors' own personal experiences. Some of the items are common sense. Regardless of their source, these stress busting activities will help you center your attention on developing a posture of expectancy and receptivity as you make an effort to keep your stress in check.

Breathe Deeply: Deep breathing is a basic technique for relaxation. Breathing slowly and deeply can help turn off stress and turn on peaceful feelings. Find a place where you can sit comfortably. Close your eyes. Inhale slowly and deeply through your nose until you have filled your stomach cavity as full as possible. Purse your lips and exhale slowly. Try doing this activity for five minutes.

Stretch: Muscle tension is a common reaction to stress. Here are some common stretches you can do at home or at work:

- Neck Stretch—while standing or sitting up straight, gently tip your head to the left, hold for 30 seconds, and then return to center. Do the same on the right side.

- Side Stretch—with your feet comfortably apart and right hand on your hip, reach your left arm overhead and stretch to the right side. Hold for 30 seconds, and then switch sides.

- Chest and Back Stretch—while standing, clasp your hands behind you, arms straight, and then lift your arms up slightly. Hold for 30 seconds. Next, clasp your hands in front of you. Rotate your shoulder, reaching as far forward as you can. Hold for 30 seconds.

- Progressive Muscular Relaxation— this 15-minute technique can help make you aware of the difference between tension and relaxation. The process is to tighten the muscle, release the tension, and then feel the difference. Settle back comfortably, either sitting or lying down. Clench your left fist. Clench it tightly and study the tension in the hand and in the forearm. Notice how it feels. Hold the tension for a few seconds. And now relax the left hand. Notice the difference between tension and relaxation. Do this with the right hand and every major muscle group of your body. You can start with your hands or move from head to toe.

Exercise: Physically active people handle stress better than those who are not active. Make time in your schedule for regular exercise. Choose an aerobic activity you can do 20-30 minutes every other day. Walking, running, swimming, and bicycling are all excellent choices. Give yourself five minutes of warm-up and five minutes of cool-down each session. Do it with friends who can help you keep your commitment, or do it alone and use the time for reflection.

Rest: A well-rested body is more resistant to stress. Try getting to bed at a reasonable hour, especially if you're under stress. Master the art of getting ready for bed. Do something relaxing before bedtime, such as taking a peaceful walk, a warm bath, a warm drink. Try to let go of the trouble of the day. As you lie down, visualize your body restoring itself with slumber.

Find Peace: Take time to fill your spiritual reservoir each day. Different things work for different people. Some fill their reservoir through prayer, meditation, thought, or pondering inspirational writings. Others fill it through admiring the beauties of nature or gazing into a star-filled sky. Do what brings you peace.

Listen to Your Body: Pay attention to what the voice of your body is telling you. The body speaks to us in many ways: by headaches, stiff necks, high blood pressure, or an upset stomach. When you "hear" these messages, you may be pushing yourself too hard. Slow down. Relax.

Think Before You Eat: Some of us use food in unhealthy ways when we are under stress. Ask yourself how you view food. Do you view eating as a way to alleviate stress? Do you eat because you are bored? If your answer is yes, try to find more positive ways to fill your empty hours. Try reading, exercise, visiting friends, taking kids on an outing, or a hobby.

TIPS FOR SPIRITUAL CARE OF DEMENTIA PATIENTS

Rev. Janet Aldrich[130] has offered a number of suggestions for nurturing spirituality: Realize that the Alzheimer's patient is still a whole person who can respond to sensory imagery, music, art, and religious ritual or symbol. Dementia patients seem to appreciate the presence of a caring visitor, listening to familiar bible verses or devotional materials, or singing familiar hymns. Attending worship services geared toward their level of cognitive impairment can create a sense of connectedness for these individuals. Since long-term memory is retained the longest, patients may enjoy reminiscing or telling their life story.

For clergy, wearing traditional vestments, and if possible, carrying a Bible, prayer book, hymnal, rosary, cross or other religious item can serve as memory "cues." Design worship experiences which are rich with sensory imagery, art, music, and religious ritual and symbol. Always identify yourself; greet the resident by name, and smile. If the patient is seated in a wheel chair, kneel down so that you are at his/her level. Use touch, when appropriate. Speak slowly and clearly, but not necessarily loudly. Face the resident when you speak and make eye contact. Use simple direct language. Ask if it is a good time for a visit (avoid mealtimes; some residents are more alert in the morning). Because of chronic fatigue and brief attention spans of persons with dementia, shorter visits usually work best.

Watch for non-verbal or behavior cues of discomfort, hunger, or thirst. Choose a quite place to talk with a minimum of noise and distractions. Ask permission to turn off television or radio. If the resident is sitting in a common area, ask if it would be okay to visit in his/her room instead. (Group visits can be confusing and increase agitation). Do not talk about the resident to others when he/she is present. Be attentive to the physical environment: room temperature (not too hot, not too cold) and lighting (avoid glare). Listen with patience, empathy, and understanding. Do not appear "rushed" by fidgeting or looking at your watch. Some residents speak very slowly and may have word-finding difficulties. Resist the temptation to "rush in" and complete the sentence for the resident. Affirm and acknowledge whatever feelings the resident is experiencing. Respond to the emotions expressed rather than the words. Do not try to deny or deflect negative emotions or attempt to "cheer up" the resident. Do not attempt to argue with the resident or try to "correct" or orient him/her to the present reality. (For example, it is not helpful to tell a resident who is looking for her mother that her mother died thirty years ago!). Such reality orientation will often increase the resident's level of anxiety.

Use validation techniques and listen for the feelings behind the statement. Try not to take rude statements or inappropriate language personally. Remember that such behavior is a manifestation of the disease. Become familiar with the Stages of Alzheimer's disease (mild, moderate and severe) so that you can recognize the kinds of behaviors which may be exhibited at each stage of the illness. If a care recipient experiences a "catastrophic reaction" in your presence, stay calm, speak quietly and reassuringly and try to distract the anxious resident. Engage a nurse or other medical professional for assistance, if one is nearby.

Do not become angry yourself in response to the outburst or try to restrain the person. If you notice that a resident looks ill or seems much more confused or anxious than usual, it is a good idea to notify medical personnel. The resident may be experiencing symptoms of a physical illness over and above those typical in dementia.

Bibliography

About Dementia. "Dementia Definition." Website of the More Focus Group. 31 May 2008 <http://www.about-dementia.com/articles/about-dementia/index.php>

Adler, Alfred. *Understanding Human Nature: The Psychology of Personality*. Oneworld Publications, 2009.

Aldrich, Janet. Chaplain, Presbyterian Homes, Evanston, IL. Personal email communication, March 2008.

Alzheimer's Association. *Official National Website*. 16 Mar. 2008 <www.alz.org >

Alzheimer's Foundation of America. 23 Apr. 2010 <http://www.alzfdn.org/>

Alzheimer's Solutions. 21 Aug. 2009 <http://alzheimersolutions.stores.yahoo.net/index.html>

American Psychiatric Association. *Diagnostic and Statistical Manual of Mental Disorders*, 4th ed., text revision (DSM- IV-TR). Washington D.C.: Author, 2000.

Anandarajah, Gowri and Ellen Hight. "Spirituality and Medical Practice: Using the HOPE Questions as a Practical Tool for Spiritual Assessment." *American Family Physician* 63, no. 1 (2001): 81-89.

Anonymous. "Take Stock Of Successes, Avoid Compassion Fatigue." *Hospital Case Management* 15, no. 2 (2007): 19-20.

Answers.com. 26 Jul 2008 <Answers.com at http://www.answers.com/topic/mental-health)>

Banks, R. "Health and Spiritual Dimensions: Relationships and Implications for Professional Preparation Programs." *Journal of School Health* 50 (1980): 195-202.

Becvar, Dorothy S. "The Impact on the Family Therapist of A Focus on Death, Dying, and Bereavement." *Journal of Marital & Family Therapy* 29, no. 4 (2003): 469-77.

Carey, Mary Elaine, PhD. Professor Emeritus, Department of Nursing, University of Oklahoma. Email correspondence, March 29, 2008.

Chao, Shu-Yuan, Hsing-Yuan Liu, Chiu-Yen Wu, Suh-Fen Jin, Tsung-Lan Chu, Tzu-Shin Huang, and Clark, Mary Jo. "The Effects of Group Reminiscence Therapy On Depression, Self Esteem, and Life Satisfaction of Elderly Nursing Home Residents." *Journal of Nursing Research* 14, no. 1 (2006): 36-45.

Chao, Shu-Yuan, Chaio-Rung Chen, Hsing-Yuan Liu, and Clark, Mary Jo. "Meet the Real Elders: Reminiscence Links Past and Present." *Journal of Clinical Nursing* 17, no. 19 (2008): 2647-53.

Collins, S. and A. Long. "Working with the Psychological Effects of Trauma: Consequences for Mental Health-Care Workers--A Literature Review." *Journal of Psychiatric & Mental Health Nursing* 10, no. 4 (2003):417-24.

Dang, Stuti, Amit Badiye, and Geetanjali Kelkar. "The Dementia Caregiver—A Primary Care Approach." *Southern Medical Journal* 101, no. 12 (2008):1246-51.

Dementia Facts and Statistics: Present and Future, *Articlesbase* 15 Aug. 2008 <http://www.articlesbase.com/anti-aging-articles/dementia-facts-and-statistics-present-and-future-523568.html>

Duncan, Stephen F. "50 Stress Busting Ideas for Your Well-being." Montana State University Extension Service. 11 Aug. 2008 <http://www.montana.edu/wwwpb/pubs/mt200016.html>

Dunn, Susan L. "Hopelessness as a Response to Physical Illness." *Journal of Nursing Scholarship* 37, no. 2 (2005): 148 – 154.

Dunne, Tad. "Spirituality and Medical Practice: Using the HOPE Questions as a Practical Tool for Spiritual Assessment." *The Hastings Center Report* 31, no. 2 (2001): 22-26.

Engel, Beverly. *Healing Your Emotional Self: A Powerful Program to Help You Raise Your Self-Esteem, Quiet Your Inner Critic, and Overcome Your Shame.* New York: John Wiley & Sons, 2006.

Figley, Charles R. "Strangers at Home: Comment on Dirkzwager, Bramsen, Ader, and van der Ploeg." *Journal of Family Psychology* 19, no. 2 (2005):227-9.

Free Dictionary (the). Learned Helplessness. 15 Apr. 2010 <http://medical-dictionary.thefreedictionary.com/learned+helplessness>

Goldsmith, Malcolm. "Through a Glass Darkly: A Dialogue between Dementia and Faith." In *Aging, Spirituality and Pastoral Care: A Multi-National Perspective*, eds. Elizabeth MacKinlay, James W. Ellor, and Stephen Pickard. New York: Haworth Pastoral Press, 2001.

Harrand, A. G. and J. J. Bollstetter. "Developing a Community-Based Reminiscence Group For the Elderly." *Clinical Nurse Specialist* 14, no. 1 (2000): 17-22.

Hogstel, M.O., L. Cox-Curry, and C. Walker. "Caring for Older Adults: The Benefits of Informal Family Caregiving." *The Journal of Theory Construction and Testing* 9, no. 2 (2005): 55-60.

Holst, Lone, Maren Lundgren, Lutte Olsen, and Torben Ishoy. "Dire Deadlines: Coping with Dysfunctional Family Dynamics in An End-of-Life Care Setting." *International Journal of Palliative Nursing* 15, no. 1 (2009): 34-41.

Hsieh, Hsiu-Fang and Jing-Jy Wang. "Effect of Reminiscence Therapy on Depression in Older Adults: A Systematic Review." *Source International Journal of Nursing Studies* 40, no. 4 (2003):335-45.

Ingersoll, R. E. "Spirituality, Religion, and Counseling: Dimensions and Relationships." *Counseling and Values* 38 (1994): 98-111.

Joinson, C. "Coping with Compassion Fatigue." *Nursing* 22, no. 4 (1992):116, 118-9, 120. Joint Commission on Accreditation of Healthcare Organizations. *The Source* 3, no. 2 (2005): 2-7.

Jones, Ellen Davis. "Reminiscence Therapy for Older Women with Depression. Effects of Nursing Intervention Classification in Assisted-Living Long-Term Care." *Journal of Gerontological Nursing* 29, no. 7 (2003): 26-33.

Jones, Ellen Davis. "The Use of Reminiscence Therapy for the Treatment of Depression in Rural-Dwelling Older Adults." *Issues in Mental Health Nursing* 23, no. 3 (2002): 279-90.

Karlikaya, G., G. Yukse, F. Varlibas, and H. Tireli. "Caregiver Burden in Dementia: A Study in the Turkish Population." *The Internet Journal of Neurology* 4, no. 2 (2005).

Kozachik, Sharon L, Gwen Wyatt, Charles W. Given, and Barbara A. Given. "Patterns of Use of Complementary Therapies among Cancer Patients and Their Family Caregivers." *Cancer Nursing* 29, no. 2 (2006): 84-94.

Liebert, Mary Ann. "Spiritual Care during Serious Illness." *Journal of Palliative Medicine* 11, no. 6 (2008).

Liebert, Mary Ann. "What Questions Do Family Caregivers Want to Discuss with Health Care Providers in Order to Prepare for The Death of A Loved One? An Ethnographic Study of Caregivers of Patients at End of Life." *Journal of Palliative Medicine* 11, no. 3 (2008).

Lin, Yen-Chun. Yu-Tzu Dai, and Shiow-Li Hwang. "The Effect of Reminiscence on the Elderly Population: A Systematic Review." *Public Health Nursing* 20, no. 4 (2003):297-306.

Mace, N. L. and P. V. Rabins. *The 36-hour Day: A Family Guide to Caring for People with Alzheimer Disease, Other Dementias, and Memory Loss in Later Life.* 4th ed. Baltimore: Johns Hopkins University Press, 2006.

Marks, N., J. D. Lambert, and H. Choi. "Transitions to Caregiving, Gender, and Psychological Well-Being: A Prospective U.S. National Study." *Journal of Marriage and Family* 64 (2002): 657–667.

Massey, Kevin, George Fitchett, and Patricia A. Roberts. "Assessment and Diagnosis in Spiritual Care." In *Spiritual Care in Nursing Practice*, eds. Kristen L. Mauk and Nola A. Schmidt. Philadelphia, PA: Lippincott, Williams, and Wilkins, 2004.

Matsa, Rabbi Myrna. (2007). "A New Model for Disaster Chaplaincy." *Journal of Jewish Communal Service* 83, no. 1 (2007): 92-98.

Mayo Foundation for Medical Education and Research (MFMER). *Official Website*, 16 Sep. 2005 < www.mayo.edu>

McHolm, Fran. "Rx for Compassion Fatigue." *Journal of Christian Nursing* 23, no. 4 (2006):12-9.

Monnot, Marilee, Meg Brosey, and Elliot Ross. "Screening for Dementia: Family Caregiver Questionnaires Reliably Predict Dementia." *JABFP* 18, no. 4 (2005).

Moody, E. F. "Life expectancy tables." 17 April 2008 <http://www.efmoody.com/estate/lifeexpectancy.html>

Mulligan, Linda. "Overcoming Compassion Fatigue." *Kansas Nurse* 79, no. 7 (2004):1-2.

National Interfaith Coalition on Aging, 1975. "Improving the Lives of Older Americans." 26 Mar. 2010 <http://www.ncoa.org/>

Nhat Hanh, Thich. *Living Buddha Living Christ*. New York: Riverhead Books, 1995.

Ostuni, E. and M. J. Santo Pietro, *Getting Through: Communicating When Someone You Care for Has Alzheimer's Disease*. Princeton Junction, NJ: The Speech Bin, 1986.

Parks, Susan Mockus and Karen D. Novielli, "A Practical Guide to Caring for Caregivers," Thomas Jefferson University Hospital, Philadelphia, Pennsylvania. *American Family Physician,* December 15, 2000. 21 Aug 2009 <http://www.aafp.org/afp/20001215/contents.html>

Perese, Eris Field, Maria Rohloff Simon, and Emily Ryan. "Promoting Positive Student Clinical Experiences with Older Adults through Use of Group Reminiscence Therapy." *Journal of Gerontological Nursing* 34, no. 12 (2008): 46-51.

Perls, Fritz. *The Gestalt Approach and Eye Witness to Therapy*. Palo Alto, CA: Science and Behavior Books, 1973.

Pickett, M., A. M. Brennan, H. S. Greenberg, L. Licht, and J. D. Worrell. "Use of Debriefing Techniques to Prevent Compassion Fatigue in Research Teams." *Nursing Research* 43, no.4 (1994): 250-2.

Pittiglio, L. "Use of Reminiscence Therapy in Patients with Alzheimer's Disease." *Lippincott's Case Management* 5, no. 6 (2000): 216-20.

Pruyser, Paul. *The Minister as Diagnostician*. Philadelphia, PA: Westminster Press, 1976.

Redinbaugh, Ellen M, Andrew Baum, Sally Tarbell, and Robert Arnold. "End-of-Life Caregiving: What Helps Family Caregivers Cope?" *Journal of Palliative Medicine* 6, no. 6 (2003): 901-9.

Reed, Lorrie. *Spiritual Renewal: A Guide to Better Health in Your Walk with God.* Orlando, FL: Higher Life, 2009.

Restak, Robert. *The Brain Has a Mind of Its Own*. New York: Crown Publishing Group, 1993.

Richards, Marty. "Meeting the Spiritual Needs of the Cognitively Impaired." *Generations* 14, no. 4 (1990): 267-274.

Roberts, Rabbi Stephen B., Kevin J. Flannelly, Andrew J. Weaver, and Charles R. Figley, "Compassion Fatigue among Chaplains, Clergy, and Other Respondents after September 11th." *Journal of Nervous & Mental Disease* 191, no. 11 (2003): 756-8.

Rourke, Mary T. "The Behavioral Health Integrated Program, The Children's Hospital of Philadelphia. Compassion fatigue in pediatric palliative care providers." *Pediatric Clinics of North America* 54, no. 5 (2007): 631-44.

Running, Alice, Lauren Woodward Tolle, and Deb Girard. "Ritual: The Final Expression of Care." *International Journal of Nursing Practice* 14, no. 4 (2008): 303-7.

Russell, Laura. "Posttraumatic Stress Disorder DSM-IV™ Diagnosis & Criteria -- 309.81" *Posttraumatic Stress Disorder*. 3 Jul. 2008 <http://www.mental-health-today.com/ptsd/dsm.htm>

Sabo, Brenda M. "Compassion Fatigue and Nursing Work: Can We Accurately Capture the Consequences of Caring Work?" *International Journal of Nursing Practice* 12, no. 3 (2006): 136-42.

Salston, Mary Dale and Charles R. Figley. "Secondary Traumatic Stress Effects of Working with Survivors of Criminal Victimization." *Journal of Traumatic Stress* 16, no. 2 (2003): 167-74.

Sanders, Sara, Carol H. Ott, Sheryl T. Kelber, and Patricia Noonan. "The Experience of High Levels of Grief in Caregivers of Persons with Alzheimer's Disease and Related Dementia." *Death Studies*, 32, no. 6 (2008):495 – 523.

Schulman, Alan and Laura C. Hanson. "Needs of the Dying in Nursing Homes." *Journal of Palliative Medicine* 5, no. 6 (2002): 895-901.

Scott A Murray, Marilyn Kendall , Kirsty Boyd, Allison Worth, and T. Fred Benton. "Exploring the spiritual needs of people dying of lung cancer or heart failure: a prospective qualitative interview study of patients and their carers." *Palliative Medicine* 18, no. 1 (2004): 39-45.

Seligman, M. E. P. "Why is there so much depression today?" In *Contemporary Psychoanalytical Approaches to Depression* (pp. 1-9), ed. R. E. Ingram. New York: Plenum, 1990.

Smith, Laurent. "Thirteen Million Baby Boomers Care for Ailing Parents, 25% Live with Parents," *Senior Journal.com.* 23 April 2010 from < http://seniorjournal.com/NEWS/Boomers/5-10-19BoomersCare4Parents.htm>

Spector, A., M. Orrell, S. Davies, and R. T. Woods. "Reminiscence therapy for dementia." *Cochrane Database of Systematic Reviews* (4):CD001120, 2000.

Stevens-Guille, Betty. "Compassion Fatigue: Who Cares for the Caregivers? The key to recovery." *Alberta RN* 59, no. 7 (2003): 18-9.

Stokes, Shirlee and Susan E. Gordon. "Common Stressors Experienced By the Well Elderly. Clinical Implications." *Journal of Gerontological Nursing* 29, no. 5 (2003): 38-46.

Stoppain.org. 21 Aug 2009 <http://www.netofcare.org/default.asp>

Tarlow, Barbara J., Stephen R. Wisniewski, Steven H. Belle, Mark Rubert, Marcia G. Ory, and Dolores Gallagher-Thompson. "Positive Aspects of Caregiving." *Research on Aging* 26, no. 4 (2004): 429-453.

University of Oklahoma Health Sciences Center. "Dementia Facts and statistics present and future." Available from https://webmail.ouhsc.edu/owa/redir.aspx?C=5ad80 f3eb5734cddb75df430190ea81b&URL=http%3a%2 f%2fwww.articlesbase.com%2fanti-aging-articles%2fdementia-facts-and-statistics-present-and-future-523568.html

Weil, Andrew. *Spontaneous Healing.* New York: Ballantine Books, 1995.

Wikipedia. Compassion Fatigue. 15 April 2010 <http://en.wikipedia.org/wiki/compassion-fatigue>

Wikipedia. Learned Helplessness. 23 April 2010 <http://medical-dictionary.thefreedictionary.com/learned+helplessness>

Wikipedia. Self-esteem. 15 April 2010 <http://en.wikipedia.org/wiki/Self-esteem>

Wilson, Karen E. "Are you a help-aholic? How to avoid compassion fatigue." *Journal of Christian Nursing* 20, no. 2 (2003): 23-4.

Woods, B., A. Spector, C. Jones, M. Orrell, and S. Davies. "Reminiscence Therapy For Dementia." In *The Cochrane Library,* no. 2, 2006. Chichester: John Wiley & Sons.

Wright, Bob. "Compassion Fatigue: How to Avoid It." *Palliative Medicine* 18, no. 1 (2004): 3-4.

Zastrow, Charles. *Introduction to Social Work and Social Welfare: Empowering People.* 9th ed. Belmont, CA: Thomson Higher Education, 2008.

REFERENCES

1 E. F. Moody, "Life expectancy tables," 17 April 2008 <http://www.efmoody.com/estate/lifeexpectancy.html>

2 Alzheimer's Foundation of America, "About Alzheimer's: Statistics," 17 April 2010 <http://www.alzfdn.org/AboutAlzheimers/statistics.html>

3 Stuti Dang, Amit Badiye, and Geetanjali Kelkar. "The Dementia Caregiver—A Primary Care Approach," *Southern Medical Journal* 101, no. 12 (2008):1246-51.

4 Stuti Dang et al., "Dementia Caregiver."

5 Stuti Dang et al., "Dementia Caregiver."

6 Alan Schulman and Laura C. Hanson, "Needs of the Dying in Nursing Homes," *Journal of Palliative Medicine* 5, no. 6 (2002): 895-901.

7 Mary Ann Liebert, "What Questions Do Family Caregivers Want to Discuss with Health Care Providers in Order to Prepare for The Death of A Loved One? An Ethnographic Study of Caregivers of Patients at End of Life," *Journal of Palliative Medicine* 11, no. 3 (2008).

8 Sara Sanders, Carol H. Ott, Sheryl T. Kelber, and Patricia Noonan, "The Experience of High Levels of Grief in Caregivers of Persons with Alzheimer's Disease and Related Dementia," *Death Studies* 32, no. 6 (July 2008): 495 – 523.

9 Sanders et al., "High levels of Grief."

10 Sanders et al., "High levels of Grief."

11 Sanders et al., "High levels of Grief."

12 Sanders et al., "High levels of Grief."

13 About Dementia, "Dementia Definition," *Website of the More Focus Group*. 31 May 2008 <http://www.aboutdementia.com/articles/about-dementia/index.php>

14 Malcolm Goldsmith, "Through a Glass Darkly: A Dialogue Between Dementia and Faith," in *Aging, Spirituality and Pastoral Care: A Multi-National Perspective*, eds. Elizabeth MacKinlay, James W. Ellor, and Stephen Pickard (New York: Haworth Pastoral Press, 2001), 130.

15 American Psychiatric Association, *Diagnostic and Statistical Manual of Mental Disorders, Fourth Edition, Text Revision (DSM- IV-TR)*, (Washington D.C., 2000).

16 Dementia Facts and Statistics: Present and Future, *Articlesbase*, August 15, 2008.
17 American Psychiatric Association, *(DSM- IV-TR)*. Washington D.C., 2000.
18 Alzheimer's Association, *Official National Website*, 16 March 2008 <www.alz.org>
19 Alzheimer's Assn., 2008.
20 Alzheimer's Assn., 2008.
21 Alzheimer's Assn., 2008.
22 Alzheimer's Assn., 2008.
23 Alzheimer's Assn., 2008.
24 Alzheimer's Assn., 2008.
25 Alzheimer's Assn., 2008.
26 Stuti Dang et al., "Dementia Caregiver."
27 Stuti Dang et al., "Dementia Caregiver."
28 Stuti Dang et al., "Dementia Caregiver."
29 Sanders et al., "High levels of Grief."
30 Sanders et al., "High levels of Grief."
31 Sanders et al., "High levels of Grief."
32 Sanders et al., "High levels of Grief."
33 Wikipedia, "Compassion Fatigue," 15 April, 2010 <http://en.wikipedia.org/wiki/Compassion Fatigue>
34 Lone Holst, Maren Lundgren, Lutte Olsen, and Torben Ishoy, "Dire deadlines: coping with dysfunctional family dynamics in an end-of-life care setting," *International Journal of Palliative Nursing* 15, no. 1 (2009): 34-41.
35 Alice Running, Lauren Woodward Tolle, and Deb Girard, "Ritual: the final expression of care," *International Journal of Nursing Practice* 14, no. 4 (2008): 303-7.
36 Mary T. Rourke, "The Behavioral Health Integrated Program, The Children's Hospital of Philadelphia. Compassion fatigue in pediatric palliative care providers," *Pediatric Clinics of North America* 54, no. 5 (2007): 631-44, x.
37 Brenda M. Sabo, "Compassion fatigue and nursing work: can we accurately capture the consequences of caring work?" *International Journal of Nursing Practice* 12, no. 3 (2006): 136-42.
38 Charles R. Figley, "Strangers at home: Comment on Dirkzwager, Bramsen, Ader, and van der Ploeg," *Journal of Family Psychology* 19, no. 2: (2005 Jun): 227-9.
39 Dorothy S. Becvar, "The impact on the family therapist of a focus on death, dying, and bereavement," *Journal of*

Marital & Family Therapy 29, no. 4 (2003): 469-77.

40 S. Collins and A. Long, "Working with the psychological effects of trauma: consequences for mental health-care workers--a literature review," *Journal of Psychiatric & Mental Health Nursing* 10, no. 4 (2003): 417-24.

41 Salston, Mary Dale and Charles R. Figley, "Secondary traumatic stress effects of working with survivors of criminal victimization, *Journal of Traumatic Stress* 16, no. 2 (2003): 167-74.

42 The following articles offer a good overview of the concept of compassion fatigue with preventive strategies identified. C. Joinson, "Coping with compassion fatigue., *Nursing* 22, no. 4 (1992): 116, 118-9, 120; Fran McHolm, "Rx for compassion fatigue," *Journal of Christian Nursing* 23, no. 4 (2006): 12-9; quiz 20-1; Linda Mulligan, "Overcoming compassion fatigue," *Kansas Nurse* 79, no 7: (2004):1-2; M. Brennan, A. M. Pickett, H. S. Greenberg, L. Licht, and J. D. Worrell, "Use of debriefing techniques to prevent compassion fatigue in research teams," *Nursing Research* 43, no. 4 (1994): 250-2; Rabbi Stephen B. Roberts, Kevin J. Flannelly, Andrew J. Weaver, and Charles R. Figley, "Compassion fatigue among chaplains, clergy, and other respondents after September 11th," *Journal of Nervous & Mental Disease* 191, no. 11: (2003): 756-8; Betty Stevens-Guille, "Compassion fatigue: who cares for the caregivers? The key to recovery," *Alberta RN* 59, no. 7 (2003): 18-9; Karen E. Wilson, "Are you a help-aholic? How to avoid compassion fatigue," *Journal of Christian Nursing* 20, no. 2 (2003): 23-4; Bob Wright, "Compassion fatigue: how to avoid it," *Palliative Medicine* 18, no. 1 (2004): 3-4.

43 Alzheimer's Solutions. 21 Aug 2009 <http://alzheimersolutions.stores.yahoo.net/index.html>

44 Stuti Dang et al., "Dementia Caregiver."

45 Alzheimer's Solutions. 21 Aug 2009 <http://alzheimersolutions.stores.yahoo.net/index.html>

46 Susan Mockus Parks and Karen D. Novielli, "A Practical Guide to Caring for Caregivers," Thomas Jefferson University Hospital, Philadelphia, Pennsylvania, *American Family Physician* December 15, 2000, 21 Aug 2009 <http://www.aafp.org/afp/20001215/contents.html>

47 G. Karlikaya, G. Yukse, F. Varlibas, and H. Tireli, "Caregiver Burden in Dementia: A Study in the Turkish

Population," *The Internet Journal of Neurology* 4, no. 2 (2005).
48 Karlikaya et al., "Caregiver Burden in Dementia."
49 Stuti Dang et al., "Dementia Caregiver."
50 Stuti Dang et al., "Dementia Caregiver."
51 Sanders et al., "High levels of Grief."
52 Stuti Dang et al., "Dementia Caregiver."
53 Stuti Dang et al., "Dementia Caregiver."
54 Stuti Dang et al., "Dementia Caregiver."
55 Laurent Smith, "Thirteen Million Baby Boomers Care for Ailing Parents, 25% Live with Parents," *Senior Journal.com* , 23 April 2010 < http://seniorjournal.com/NEWS/Boomers/5-10-19BoomersCare4Parents.htm>
56 Stuti Dang et al., "Dementia Caregiver."
57 Sanders et al., "High levels of Grief."
58 Sanders et al., "High levels of Grief."
59 M. O. Hogstel et al., "Caring for Older Adults."
60 M. O. Hogstel et al., "Caring for Older Adults."
61 M. O. Hogstel et al., "Caring for Older Adults."
62 M. O. Hogstel et al., "Caring for Older Adults."
63 M. O. Hogstel et al., "Caring for Older Adults."
64 Marilee Monnot, Meg Brosey, and Elliott Ross, "Screening for Dementia: Family Caregiver Questionnaires Reliably Predict Dementia." *JABFP* 18, no. 4 (2005).
65 See N. L. Mace and P. V. Rabins, *The 36-hour day: A family guide to caring for people with Alzheimer disease, other dementias, and memory loss in later life* (4th ed.) (Baltimore, MD: Johns Hopkins University Press, 2006).
Also see E. Ostuni, E. and M. J. Santo Pietro, *Getting through: Communicating when someone you care for has Alzheimer's disease* (Princeton Junction, NJ: The Speech Bin, 1986).
66 Alzheimer's Association. *Official National Website.* 16 March 2008 <www.alz.org >
67 Susan L. Dunn, "Hopelessness as a Response to Physical Illness," *Journal of Nursing Scholarship* 37, no. 2 (2005); 148-154.
68 Wikipedia. Learned Helplessness. 23 April 2010 < http://medicaldictionary.thefreedictionary.com/learned+helplessness>
69 Wikipedia. Self-Esteem. 23 April 2010 <http://en.wikipedia.org/wiki/Self-esteem>
70 Malcolm Goldsmith, "Through a Glass Darkly: A Dialogue Between Dementia and Faith," in *Aging, Spirituality*

and Pastoral Care: A Multi-National Perspective, eds. Elizabeth MacKinlay, James W. Ellor, and Stephen Pickard,
(New York: Haworth Pastoral Press, 2001), 130.

[71] B. Woods, A. Spector, C. Jones, M. Orrell, and S. Davies, "Reminiscence therapy for dementia," *Cochrane Database of Systematic Reviews,* Issue (2):CD001120, 2005.

[72] Yen-Chun Lin, Yu-Tzu Dai, and Shiow-Li Hwang, "The effect of reminiscence on the elderly population: a systematic review," *Public Health Nursing* 20, no. 4 (2003): 297-306.

[73] B. Woods, A. Spector, and C. Jones et al. "Reminiscence therapy for dementia," *The Cochrane Library,* Issue 2, 2006.

[74] Eris Field Perese, Maria Rohloff Simon, and Emily Ryan, "Promoting positive student clinical experiences with older adults through use of group reminiscence therapy," *Journal of Gerontological Nursing* 34, no. 12 (2008): 46-51.

[75] Erise Field Perese et al., "Promoting positive student clinical experiences."

[76] Shu-Yuan Chao, Chaio-Rung Chen, Hsing-Yuan Liu, and Mary Jo Clark, "Meet the real elders: reminiscence links past and present," *Journal of Clinical Nursing* 17, no. 19 (2008): 2647-53.

[77] Sharon L. Kozachik, Gwen Wyatt, Charles W. Given, and Barbara A. Given, "Patterns of use of complementary therapies among cancer patients and their family caregivers," *Cancer Nursing* 29, no. 2 (2006): 84-94.

[78] Shu-Yuan Chao, Hsing-Yuan Liu, Chiu-Yen Wu, Suh-fen Jin, Tsung-Lan Chu, Tzu-Shin Huang, and Mary Jo Clark, "The effects of group reminiscence therapy on depression, self esteem, and life satisfaction of elderly nursing home residents," *Journal of Nursing Research* 14, no 1 (2006): 36-45.

[79] The objective of the review is to assess the effects of reminiscence therapy for older people with dementia and their care-givers. Search strategy: The trials were identified from a search of the Specialized Register of the Cochrane Dementia and Cognitive Improvement Group on 4 May 2004 using the term "reminiscence."

[80] Ellen Davis Jones, "Reminiscence therapy for older women with depression. Effects of nursing intervention classification in assisted-living long-term care," *Journal of Gerontological Nursing* 29, no. 7 (2003): 26-33; quiz 56-7.

81 Mary E. Carey, personal email communication, 2008.

82 Gowri Anandarajah and Ellen Hight, "Spirituality and Medical Practice: Using the HOPE Questions as a
Practical Tool for Spiritual Assessment," *American Family Physician* 63, no. 1 (2001): 81-89.

83 Fritz Perls, *The Gestalt Approach and Eye Witness to Therapy* (Palo Alto, CA: Science and Behavior Books,
1973).

84 Fritz Perls, *The Gestalt Approach and Eye Witness to Therapy*. See also Alfred Adler, *Understanding Human
Nature: The Psychology of Personality* (Oneworld Publications, 2009); American Psychiatric Association.
Diagnostic and Statistical Manual of Mental Disorders, 4th ed., Text Revision (DSM- IV-TR). Washington D.C.,
2000.

85 American Psychiatric Association. *(DSM- IV-TR)*. Washington D.C., 2000.

86 M. E. P. Seligman, "Why is there so much depression today?" In *Contemporary psychoanalytical approaches to
depression* (pp. 1-9), ed. R. E. Ingram (New York: Plenum, 1990).

87 R. Banks, "Health and Spiritual Dimensions: Relationships and Implications for Professional Preparation
Programs," *Journal of School Health* 50 (1980): 196.

88 R. E. Ingersoll, "Spirituality, Religion, and Counseling: Dimensions and Relationships," *Counseling and Values*
38 (1994): 98-111.

89 Banks, 1980; Ingersoll, 1994.

90 Robert Restak, *The Brain Has a Mind of Its Own* (New York, NY: Crown Publishing Group, 1993), 4.

91 Restak, *The Brain,* 4.

92 Restak, *The Brain*, 12.

93 Beverly Engel, *Healing Your Emotional Self: A Powerful Program to Help You Raise Your Self-Esteem, Quiet
Your Inner Critic, and Overcome Your Shame* (New York: John Wiley & Sons, 2006), 146.

94 Engel, *Healing Your Emotional Self,* 146.

95 Andrew Weil, *Spontaneous Healing* (New York: Ballantine Books, 1995).

96 Andrew Weil, *Spontaneous Healing,* 1995, p. 126.

97 Gowri Anandarajah and Ellen Hight, "Spirituality and Medical Practice: Using the HOPE Questions as a Practical
Tool for Spiritual Assessment," *American Family Physician* 63, no. 1 (2001):81-89.

98 Lorrie Reed, *Spiritual Renewal: A Guide to Better Health in Your Walk with God* (Orlando, FL: Higher Life, 2009).
99 Gowri Anandarajah and Ellen Hight, "Spirituality and Medical Practice."
100 Mayo Foundation for Medical Education and Research.
101 Marty Richards, "Meeting the Spiritual Needs of the Cognitively Impaired," *Generations* 14, no. 4 (1990): 267-274.
102 Gowri Anandarajah and Ellen Hight, "Spirituality and Medical Practice."
103 Sanders et al., "High levels of Grief."
104 Tad Dunne, "Spirituality and Medical Practice: Using the HOPE Questions as a Practical Tool for Spiritual Assessment ," *The Hastings Center Report*, 31, no. 2 (Mar. - Apr., 2001):22-26.
105 Murray A. Scott, Marilyn Kendall, Kirsty Boyd, Allison Worth, and T. Fred Benton, "Exploring the spiritual needs of people dying of lung cancer or heart failure: a prospective qualitative interview study of patients and their carers," *Palliative Medicine* 18 (2004): 39-45.
106 Murray A. Scott et al.
107 Mayo Foundation for Medical Education and Research.
108 Gowri Anandarajah and Ellen Hight, "Spirituality and Medical Practice."
109 Janet Aldrich personal email communication, 2008.
110 Aldrich, 2008.
111 Joint Commission on Accreditation of Healthcare Organizations, *The Source* 3, no. 2 (2005): 2-7.
112 Gowri Anandarajah and Ellen Hight, "Spirituality and Medical Practice."
113 Stuti Dang et al., "Dementia Caregiver."
114 Malcolm Goldsmith, 2001, 130.
115 Aldrich, 2008.
116 Stuti Dang et al., "Dementia Caregiver."
117 Ellen M. Redinbaugh, Andrew Baum, Sally Tarbell, and Robert Arnold. "End-of-Life Caregiving: What Helps Family Caregivers Cope?" *Journal of Palliative Medicine* 6, no. 6 (2003):901-9.
118 Ellen M. Redinbaugh et al., "End-of-Life Caregiving"
119 Stuti Dang et al., "Dementia Caregiver."
120 Stuti Dang et al., "Dementia Caregiver."
121 Mayo Foundation for Medical Education and Research.

[122] Mayo Foundation for Medical Education and Research.
[123] Mayo Foundation for Medical Education and Research.
[124] Mary E. Carey, personal email communication, 2008.
[125] Kevin Massey, George Fitchett, and Patricia A. Roberts, "Assessment and Diagnosis in Spiritual Care," in *Spiritual Care in Nursing Practice*, eds. Kristen L. Mauk and Nola A. Schmidt (Philadelphia, PA: Lippincott, Williams, and Wilkins, 2004).
[126] Massey, Fitchett, and Roberts, 2004.
[127] Paul Pruyser, *The Minister as Diagnostician* (Philadelphia, PA: Westminster Press, 1976).
[128] From "Stoppain.org retrieved 21 Aug 2009 from http://www.netofcare.org/default.asp
[129] Stephen F. Duncan, "50 Stress Busting Ideas for Your Well-being," Montana State University Extension Service, 11 Aug. 2008 <http://www.montana.edu/wwwpb/pubs/mt200016.html>
[130] Aldrich, 2008.

www.ingramcontent.com/pod-product-compliance
Lightning Source LLC
LaVergne TN
LVHW051505070426
835507LV00022B/2941